D0579029

STEALTH
HEALTH

Also by Evelyn Tribole

HEALTHY HOMESTYLE DESSERTS

INTUITIVE EATING (COAUTHOR)

HEALTHY HOMESTYLE COOKING

EATING ON THE RUN

Evelyn Tribole, M.S., R.D.

Photographs by Sally Ann Ullman

STEALTH
HEALTH

How to Sneak

Nutrition

Painlessly

into Your Diet

VIKING

VIKING
Published by the Penguin Group
Penguin Putnam Inc., 375 Hudson Street,
New York, New York 10014, U.S.A.
Penguin Books Ltd, 27 Wrights Lane, London W8 5TZ, England
Penguin Books Australia Ltd, Ringwood, Victoria, Australia
Penguin Books Canada Ltd, 10 Alcorn Avenue,
Toronto, Ontario, Canada M4V 3B2
Penguin Books (N.Z.) Ltd, 182–190 Wairau Road,
Auckland 10, New Zealand
Penguin India, 210 Chiranjiv Tower, 43 Nehru Place,
New Delhi, 11009 India

Penguin Books Ltd, Registered Offices:
Harmondsworth, Middlesex, England

First published in 1998 by Viking Penguin,
a member of Penguin Putnam Inc.

1   3   5   7   9   10   8   6   4   2

LIBRARY OF CONGRESS CATALOGING-IN-PUBLICATION DATA
Tribole, Evelyn, 1959–
Stealth health : how to sneak nutrition painlessly into your diet / Evelyn Tribole : photographs by
Sally Ann Ullman.
p.   cm.
Includes index.
ISBN 0-670-87499-X
1. Nutrition.   2. Health.   3. Low-fat-diet—Recipes.   4. Low-calorie diet—Recipes.   I. Title.
RA784.T753   1998
613.2—dc21   98-8041

This book is printed on acid-free paper.
∞

Sally Ann Ullman—Photographer
Lari Robling—Food Stylist
Terry Ruhl—Prop Stylist
Prop Credits—Domostyle/Home Place—Buckingham, PA

Printed in the United States of America
Set in Garamond Light
Designed by Kathryn Parise

To my best friend, Jeff

ACKNOWLEDGMENTS

One of the best parts of completing a book is getting the opportunity to thank everyone. I am especially grateful to:

Michelle Marin, who spent hours at the library faithfully gathering my research.

Dawn Drzal—a delightful editor, whose enthusiasm for this project kept the wind in my writing sails.

David Smith—my literary agent and champion. I feel fortunate to have an agent whom I trust and respect.

I am indebted to my personal team of taste testers—a cadre of neighbors, friends, and family, who would drop everything at a moment's notice to taste my new creations. Thank you Jim and Margie Jakowatz, Alan and Linaya Pavlish, Patty and Chris Peck, and to my special troubleshooter and sister, Elaine Roberts.

I am thankful to Lari Robling, who put my recipes through another round of testing and offered useful feedback. I appreciated her attention to detail and her shared passion for these recipes to be stellar. To Sally Ullman, photographer and Terry Ruhl, prop stylist, for making the *Stealth* recipes come alive (and to Lari, once again, for her skillful food styling for the photos).

I offer special thanks and love to my family, Jeff, Connor, and Krystin, for patiently putting up with me.

CONTENTS

1   Vegetable Kingdom   9

This chapter is targeted to the person who either dislikes vegetables or simply has difficulty getting them into the diet. Recipes include Sunburst Soup and Pumpkin Pie Shake.

2   Coming to Fruition   39

This chapter is geared to the person who has trouble getting enough fruit into the diet. Recipes include Paradise Shake and Strawberries and Cream Pie.

3 Calcium Quota   63

This chapter is aimed at the individual who either dislikes milk or has difficulty consuming it. He or she may avoid milk for ethical or other reasons, but does not make an effort to consume other high-calcium foods. These calcium-rich recipes include Cheesy Stuffed Shells and Deep Chocolate Pudding.

4 The Joy of Soy   87

Exciting research has shown that adding soy into your diet can reduce cholesterol levels and alleviate the side effects of menopause. Since most Americans have not been exposed to tofu or soy products, they are often afraid to eat tofu or soy. Recipes include Toasted Tacos Ole and Chocolate Marble Cheesecake.

5 Full of Beans   113

Beans are the unsung heroes of nutrition—loaded with folic acid, fiber, and protein. Recipes include Enchilada Bake and Dark Fudge Brownies.

6 Fiber Imbiber   135

This chapter will concentrate on how to get fiber from whole grains. Recipes include Jeff's Thick-Crust Bread-Machine Pizza and Cinnayum Rolls.

7 Iron Men and Maidens   169

Iron deficiency is the number one nutrition problem in children and a key problem for women in the childbearing years. Iron-rich recipes include Manhattan (Red) Clam Chowder and Spiced Gingerbread.

8 Trimming the Fat   195

This chapter includes recipes that illustrate key fat-cutting techniques that still keep that wonderful mouth-feel and flavor, including Onion Rings and Sweet and Sour Pork.

STEALTH HEALTH

Introduction

Have you ever loaded up on a bunch of fresh vegetables only to have them sit lonely and wilted in your fridge by the end of the week? Or perhaps you've heard the good news about soy foods, but the idea of tofu and all its cousins makes you shudder.

Whether you are a devout vegetable hater or just have trouble eating the foods that are "good for you," I have created *Stealth Health* to help you (and perhaps your family or loved ones) sneak nutrition into familiar and nonthreatening recipes such as:

• Chocolate Marble Cheesecake—no one would know by looking or tasting, but there's pureed tofu in it!
• Spiced Gingerbread—made with whole wheat flour but so moist and delicious.
• Cheddar Chowder—with carrots grated so fine they look like flecks of Cheddar cheese.

I was inspired to write this book because of experiences with my family, friends, clients, and readers. One particular moment stands out. I was creating my Recipe Makeover column for *Shape* magazine and had a

1

bit of an epiphany. I was trying to lower the fat in a dessert and found that a combination of corn syrup and marshmallow creme did the job superbly. But I stepped back for a moment and asked myself . . . what am I doing? I certainly cut the fat, but I can't say that I was contributing to the nutritional welfare of readers. I started to think about all the fat-free foods and what was in them—in many cases just sugar and white flour, sans fat—not exactly a stellar example of healthful eating.

In the interest of lowering fat many of us have forgotten the big picture, that healthful eating includes whole foods, whole grains, fresh fruits and vegetables, and so on.

In my practice I have been seeing a lot of patients who eat very low-fat diets, yet their weight keeps climbing. Nutritionally their diets are usually lacking in whole grains, fruits, and vegetables. In the past (before the arrival of fat-free foods), a low-fat diet was usually healthy because you had to base your diet around fruits, vegetables, whole grains, lean meats, beans, and low-fat dairy. Ironically, with the proliferation of fat-free and reduced-fat foods (over 5600 of them), our diets are *not* improving. The latest government surveys reinforce this by showing:

• Americans are eating more calories than ever (up by an average of 300 a day)
• Actual fat gram consumption has increased for both men and women
• We repeatedly fall short in consumption of fruits, vegetables, whole grains, iron-rich foods, fiber, calcium, folic acid while we still eat too much fat!

AWESOME RESEARCH—THE WHOLE FOOD TRUTH

It has never been clearer that what you eat can make a big difference to your health. But the secret to health is not stocking up on fat-free foods or loading up on supplements. It lies in nature's special package— food. Right now research is exploding with example on example of compounds discovered in food that benefit health, yet they are not nutrients—they are phytochemicals. Phytochemicals are natural chemicals found in plant foods that have special health-enhancing abilities from fighting cancer to lowering blood cholesterol. These compounds are so promising that the National Cancer Institute has spent in excess of $20 million researching the anti-cancer potential of plant foods, and this is only one arena of preventive research. Here are just a few examples of nature's chemical soup (more examples are laced throughout the book):

- Soy foods are rich in a variety of phytochemicals, some of which are potent switches that lower cholesterol in our bodies. Other soy phytochemicals show strong anti-cancer activity and may help to alleviate PMS and menopause symptoms.
- Egallic acid, an active cancer-fighting compound, has been discovered in grapes, strawberries, and raspberries.
- A single orange has more than 170 phytochemicals.
- Whole wheat has hundreds of phytochemicals, but they are concentrated in the bran and the germ. Unfortunately, these phytos are eliminated when processed into white flour products.
- Glucorates, another cancer fighter, has been discovered in citrus, grains, tomatoes, and peppers.
- There are almost two thousand known plant pigments that not only give a beautiful rainbow of colors to our food but have been shown to protect us from disease.

Try as you might, you can't pack all this amazing stuff into a supplement! This especially holds true for all the phytochemicals yet to be discovered since the science is still new.

What to do, what to do, what to do? These days, I find that achieving a healthful diet is not usually an issue of needing more knowledge about nutrition; it's an issue of finding ways to fit these foods into your diet and lifestyle on a regular basis. (Or finding ways to painlessly sneak these foods into your recipes.)

I want to be clear, however; I'm not talking about coercive measures, just subtle flavorful ones—whether that means altering texture or presentation, or just adding a complete surprise ingredient to a familiar recipe. In fact, food-tasting demonstrations (whether at presentations, at home, or on live television) have taught me that tasting is believing. A critical key to success was and still is never to tell my taster what is in the food—to prevent taste-bud bias and preconceived notions. I am always happy to reveal my ingredients *after* someone has tasted them!

If you are worried because you are a self-proclaimed picky eater or cook for a family of them, read on!

WHAT WE CAN LEARN FROM THE PICKY EATER . . .
SURVIVAL INSTINCT

Children are naturally reluctant to eat new foods. In fact, this is so common that researchers have coined a new word for it—neophobia. Neophobia is credited with our survival (as a means of learned safety). Prehistoric people, foraging for food and eating whatever looked good, could easily drop dead if they picked the wrong plant, say a poisonous mushroom. Our natural reluctance to eat new foods minimized our risk from toxic plants. If we took a bite of a new food and had no ill consequences we gradually learned that that particular food was safe to eat. Keep this in mind when introducing new foods to children:

• Don't interpret a child's initial rejection of a new food as a permanent aversion.

• It may take eight to ten times of *tasting* a new food before it becomes accepted, according to the research of Leann L. Birch, a renowned authority on toddler eating behavior. *But merely looking at and smelling a food this many times will not lead to greater acceptance!* Therefore, we need to gently encourage our children to taste new foods.

• Keep in mind that the environment in which you have a child sample a new food is critical. Conditions need to be favorable and refrain from coercive feeding techniques.

This approach works well with adults, too. The basis of *Stealth Health* cooking is *tasting is believing.* For example, one of my favorite fat-cutting techniques is using baby food prunes in place of fat in chocolate desserts such as brownies or fudge. Before this technique caught on, people would snicker a bit and roll an eyeball or two. Until they tasted the goodie, they couldn't believe it!

Tofu is another good example. I have found that the mere mention of tofu can provoke a disdainful look. Yet if I make a delicious cheesecake (page 111) and have a person taste it (without mentioning the ingredients), I get raves. I usually win over a convert or two, or at least open someone's mind! There are many more examples throughout the recipe section of this book.

You are certainly entitled to your food preferences. I would only be concerned if these preferences knock out a whole category of food, such as all vegetables or all fruits.

ABOUT THE RECIPES

These recipes have been developed and tested by yours truly, then taste-tested by neighbors, friends, and family. After the recipes passed the initial taste test, they went through one more round of rigorous testing by an independent professional recipe tester.

Each recipe has several bits of information for your learning pleasure:

• *The Sneak*—describes how I stealthily incorporate an ingredient into a recipe. I hope it will serve as a springboard for you to try new ideas on your own.

• *Nutrition Scorecard*—provides the basic calories, fat in both grams and as a percentage of calories, carbohydrates, and cholesterol.

• *Notable Nutrient*—tells you what key nutrient is present at high levels. Please be sure to note the term % Daily Value (%DV). The %DV is a quick way to size up the nutritional value of a food without memorizing grams or carrying a calculator. The %DV number is a goal or target for the entire day. It indicates how close you are to the goal when eating one serving of a particular food.

GETTING STARTED

Each chapter stands on its own and gives the latest research on why a food or nutrient is so important. But more important, there are over a hundred recipes to help you get more of the "problem foods" into your diet. Quick nutrition research bits are also woven throughout the recipe sections.

You may want to jump around and head straight for your problem area. Take a look at the following chart, Problem Areas at a Glance, and you will see which chapter is perfect for you and you'll know where to begin.

Just remember, what counts is progress not perfection.

Problem Areas at a Glance . . . Which Are You?

Examine the traits for each problem area. If you answer yes to any of the traits your diet could probably use some improvement.

Are You a . . . ?	Traits	Then Go to:
Vegetable Hater	• Ranges from inconsistent to never eating vegetables. • Vegetables are too much of a hassle. • Noble intentions result in a refrigerator full of wilted vegetables by the end of the week. • Hates vegetables, taste and texture. • Eats less than three servings a day of vegetables. • Diet is high in fast foods.	CHAPTER 1 *Vegetable Kingdom*
Fruit Skimper	• Does not necessarily dislike fruit, but it is not eaten consistently. • Eats less than two fruit servings a day (including juice).	CHAPTER 2 *Fruit*
Milk Miser	• Chooses to avoid milk for ethical or other reasons, but does not make an effort to consume other high-calcium foods. • Dislikes the taste of milk and dairy products. • Consuming dairy results in side effects such as gas, bloating.	CHAPTER 3 *Calcium*
Soy Coy	• Soy foods such as tofu are rarely eaten, if at all. • Afraid to try soy foods.	CHAPTER 4 *Joy of Soy*
Bean Barren	• Beans are rarely eaten, if at all. • Eats beans less than three times per week.	CHAPTER 5 *Full of Beans*
Ironless	• Diet is typically low in red meats. • Diet is low in dark meat poultry. • Diet is low in dried fruits.	CHAPTER 7 *Iron*

Are You a . . . ?	Traits	Then Go to:
Fiber Depriver	• Eats highly processed foods, including a lot of packaged fat-free foods. • White flour-based foods are the staple grain in the diet (bagels, pasta, baguettes, sourdough bread). • Rarely uses whole wheat bread or whole wheat flour. • Diet is low in fruits and vegetables.	**CHAPTER 6** *Fiber Imbiber*
Fat Lover	• Loves sauces and dressings: oil-based, cream-based. • Sandwiches filled with mayonnaise. • Eats lots of fried foods and fatty snacks. • Diet is highly meat-based. • No bread goes unbuttered or undrizzled with oil.	**CHAPTER 8** *Trimming the Fat*

CHAPTER ONE

Vegetable Kingdom

Why Veggies Are *So* Important

"I wish I liked vegetables, I really do." That's what one of my clients sincerely lamented. But she's not the only one struggling.

It's no secret that vegetables are important to health, yet it's one area that Americans continually have trouble with. According to the USDA's survey on American eating habits, on any given day only one in ten Americans eats a dark green or deep yellow vegetable, while one in four munches on french fries and mashed potatoes. We're at the low end of the recommended three to five servings daily, with almost half coming from potatoes. Yet more than half the country isn't eating even that much.

PHYTO POWER

While nutritionists have touted for years the importance of vegetables, study after study demonstrates that plant foods confer health benefits *beyond* their bounty of nutrients. These beneficial compounds are called phytochemicals, and scientists have barely scratched the surface of identifying them (there are estimated to be hundreds of them) and

9

figuring out what they do exactly. Remember these are not vitamins or nutrients, but powerful plant compounds that you can get only by eating plant foods! Supplement manufacturers cannot package into a bottle compounds that have yet to be identified by scientists. Phytochemicals may be the real ally in fighting heart disease, cancer, and other diseases because of their powerful detoxifying enzymes and antioxidant abilities. Here's a glimpse of how and why.

• *Detoxification Enzymes*—help remove harmful agents from the body, akin to taking a stinger out of a bee. For example, cruciferous vegetables (cabbage vegetables and their cousins) contain indole-3-carbinol. Indole-3-carbinol has been shown to reduce potent forms of estrogen, which may help protect against estrogen-related cancers of the breast and endometrial cancer. Broccoli contains sulphorophane, which appears to be an exceptionally powerful switch that turns on several detox enzymes. Allium vegetables such as onions, leeks, and garlic are rich in sulfide phytochemicals that help the body rid itself of cancer-causing substances.

• *Phyto Antioxidant Power*—promising USDA research shows that plant foods possess natural compounds that generate antioxidant action independent of their antioxidant nutrients such as vitamin C.

Researchers measured the antioxidant power of common vegetables and fruits using a new technique called the oxygen radical absorbance capacity (ORAC). Using ORAC, researchers at Tufts University found that plant-based foods contain a natural antioxidant mixture that appears to be better than a single antioxidant nutrient (or even a mixture of nutrients). Of the vegetables, kale had the most antioxidant activity followed by beets, red bell pepper, broccoli flower, spinach, potato, sweet potato, and corn.

Keep in mind that this research took place in a pristine test tube. The next step is to find out if these results hold up in animals (and people) and to identify the specific compounds that give vegetables (and other plants) their antioxidant power. It also reinforces the fact that there's no getting around the basic mantra of "eat your veggies."

Antioxidants serve as pollution control for our body to get rid of wayward oxygen. Ironically, while oxygen is essential for life, when it is metabolized in our cells it can wreak havoc, if not properly contained, by a process called oxidation. Oxidation is the biological equivalent of rusting. Antioxidants trap the oxygen and prevent cellular rusting. For instance, if you slice open an apple and leave it out for a while, oxygen (or the process of oxidation) will turn the apple brown. But if you apply an antioxidant to the exposed apple, it will prevent the oxidation and no browning will occur. (That's why you often see recipes instructing that raw apples be soaked in orange or lemon juice; the vitamin C in these juices prevents browning.) This is a simplified version of how antioxidants protect our bodies.

Antioxidants also help prevent cell damage from attack by free radicals. Free radicals are unstable compounds generated by the body. They are like charged molecular tornados looking for something to pair up with. But in the quest of seeking and hooking up with electron buddies, they can damage anything in their path, including vital cell structures. Antioxidants are capable of scavenging and neutralizing free radicals. Many chronic diseases such as heart disease, cancer, and cataracts are believed to be caused in part by damage from oxygen or free radicals.

NUTRITIONAL GOLD MINE

Of course, we can't forget the obvious, vegetables are a rich source of important vitamins, minerals, and fiber. Imagine, just one yellow bell pepper contains five times the vitamin C of one orange. One carrot gives you twice your vitamin A needs for the day. Take a look at the two charts, Veggies Super High in Vitamin A and Veggies Super High in Vitamin C, and you'll appreciate what some vegetables can do to boost your nutrition.

Vitamin A in plants is found in the form of carotenoids. You may be familiar with the most famous carotenoid, beta-carotene. But beta-carotene is just one of six hundred carotenoids that give vegetables their deep yellow/orange color. They are also plentiful in dark green vegetables, but the vivid sunset colors are masked by the abundant chlorophyll. Only the major carotenoids, alpha-carotene, beta-carotene, and beta-cryptoxanthin can be converted to vitamin A in the body. But many carotenoids act as antioxidants. For example, lycopene, found mostly in tomatoes, has twice the antioxidant potency of beta-carotene. A large study in the United States associated high intakes of lycopene (from pizza sauce and tomatoes) with a reduced risk of prostate cancer. Lycopene or the food that contains it has also been associated with reduced risks of other cancers, including cancer of the bladder, pancreas, and digestive tract.

TURNING OVER A NEW LEAF (PREFERABLY LEAFY GREENS)

Okay, so you get the message—you need to eat vegetables. Let's see where you (or your family) stands. Just answer Yes or No to the following questions (be honest with yourself here).

1. Do you eat less than three servings each day of vegetables? (One serving is ½ cup cooked or 1 cup raw.)
2. Is your diet high in fast food and restaurant meals—more than three times a week?
3. Do you often begin the week with noble intentions and a cartful of veggies to wind up only with a refrigerator full of wilted vegetables by the end of the week?
4. Do you dislike or even (gasp) hate vegetables, their taste and texture?

Answering Yes to any of these questions poses a problem. Let's look at the solutions.

• *How Much to Eat?*—aim for an absolute minimum of three servings each day, the more the better. It doesn't have to be three different vegetables (although variety is always a great idea). For example 1½ cups of broccoli is three servings worth. Even getting into the habit of eating a vegetable with lunch and dinner will help establish a framework in which you automatically plug in your vegetable.

Research from the prominent DASH study (Dietary Approaches to Stop Hypertension) showed that increasing plant food in the diet to a minimum of eight servings from fruits and vegetables (four servings of each) in combination with eating low-fat foods lowered blood pressure within two weeks of starting the diet. The researchers estimated that if Americans ate this way there would be 27 percent fewer strokes and 15 percent less coronary heart disease.

• *Fast Food and Restaurant Meals*—if you dine frequently on fast foods it is a challenge to get a vegetable. (And please—do not count french fries as a vegetable.) Your best bet here is to include a side salad or baked potato. Or be sure to double up at the next meal. You may also want to try places like Boston Market or Koo Koo Roo, which feature many vegetable and salad side dishes.

Restaurants can be a particularly easy place to get veggies; you just need to remember to make them a priority or they could be absent by default. I find it is helpful to develop the expectation of "How am I going to get a vegetable at this meal?" If you don't, you can easily wind up with a lunch meal of a sandwich and fries sans vegetables. While salads and vegetable-based soups are great and easy ways to include vegetables, I am particularly fond of ordering an extra side of grilled vegetables. They are often not listed on the menu but are easily accommodated.

• *Good-Intentioned Veggie Eater*—you are probably someone who knows the healthy value of veggies and actually likes to eat them. Consistency is usually the issue here. Be careful that you are not falling into the perfectionism trap that goes something like this: "Fresh is best and if I don't have fresh, then I do without." A person does not usually start off the day by stating I will not eat vegetables for dinner tonight since I have no fresh produce on hand. But the belief that only fresh will do nutritionally prevents that person from exploring frozen options and even canned.

• *Vegetable Haters or Resisters*—don't give up hope (and also don't fool yourself into thinking that you can rely on a supplement to fix the deficit). The most important thing is to begin with the vegetables that you do like. Every devout vegetable hater that I've met along the way usually has a few vegetables that he or she will eat or "tolerate." Start with those—even if it means serving the same vegetable every night with dinner.

There are many ways to try vegetables or even sneak them into your diet.

Five Ways to Sneak Veggies into Meals

1. Puree a vegetable and add it to a sauce or soup. For example, see Twice-Baked Potatoes, page 28, for a clever cauliflower sneak.

2. Grate or chop a vegetable into tiny almost undetectable bits. For example, see the Cheddar Chowder, page 19, in which bits of carrot resemble flecks of Cheddar cheese.

3. Disguise a vegetable. Snipped ribbons of spinach and other leafy greens resemble herbs such as basil. For example, see Home-Style Lasagna, page 23, in which kale is disguised as basil in the spaghetti sauce.

4. Spice it up. Use strong savory flavors from chilies, garlic, and ginger to help divert the taste buds. For example, see Sunburst Soup, page 18.

5. Treat a vegetable as an integral part of a main dish rather than having it sit isolated on the plate. Or build a main dish around a vegetable. For example, see Chicken Chili Verde, page 26.

Veggies Super High in Vitamin A

These particular vegetables are packed with vitamin A, in most cases providing more than 1000 Retinol Equivalents (RE) or over 100 percent of what you need in a day.

Vegetable	Vitamin A (RE)	%DV (percent Daily Value)
Bell pepper, raw, 1	678	68
Butternut squash, 1 cup, baked	1436	144
Carrot, 1 raw	2025	202
Carrot juice, ½ cup	3159	316
Dandelion greens, 1 cup:		
raw	770	77
cooked from fresh	1229	130
Hubbard squash, 1 cup, baked	1450	145
Pumpkin, canned, ½ cup	2702	270
Spinach, 1 cup:		
raw	448	145
cooked from frozen	1756	176
cooked from fresh	1750	148
canned, drained	1878	188
Sweet Potato		
baked 1	2488	249
canned, mashed, ½ cup	1929	193
Swiss chard, cooked, 1 cup	1198	120
Turnip greens, cooked, 1 cup:		
from fresh	792	79
from frozen	1308	131

Veggies Super High in Vitamin C

These particular vegetables are packed with vitamin C, in most cases providing more than 60 milligrams or over 100 percent of what you need in a day.

Vegetable	Vitamin C milligrams	%DV (percent Daily Value)
Bell pepper		
red, 1 whole raw	141	235
green, 1 whole raw	66	110
yellow, 1 whole raw	341	568
Broccoli, 1 cup:		
raw	82	137
cooked from frozen	74	123
cooked from fresh	116	267
Brussels sprouts, 1 cup:		
cooked from frozen	97	162
cooked from fresh	71	118
Cauliflower, 1 cup:		
raw	72	120
cooked from frozen	56	93
cooked from fresh	68	113
Kale, 1 cup:		
raw	80	133
cooked from frozen	33	55
cooked from fresh	53	88
Kohlrabi, 1 cup:		
raw	87	145
cooked from fresh	89	148
Vegetable juice cocktail, 1 cup	67	112

Twenty Ways to Increase Vegetables in Your Diet

1. Remember that eating any vegetable, whether canned or frozen, is an improvement over not eating one at all.

2. Grow a vegetable garden. There's nothing like the flavor of a home-grown vegetable and kids love it. If space is limited, try planting in a pot of soil.

3. Change the texture of vegetables from cooked and soft to raw and crunchy. For example, instead of serving cooked carrots with a meal, don't be afraid to offer crisp raw carrots instead.

4. Adorn a favorite food with vegetables. Try topping your pizza with chopped bell peppers.

5. Don't be afraid to add a little butter or margarine if that makes the difference between eating vegetables or not.

6. Enhance veggies with fresh herbs—garlic, ginger, and basil can do wonders.

7. Steam in a flavorful broth such as chicken stock or vegetable broth.

8. Throw some vegetables on the grill, either whole or large skewer pieces.

9. Double your normal portion for vegetables.

10. Try vegetable or tomato juice for a beverage—it counts as a vegetable serving.

11. Try one new vegetable or vegetable-based recipe each week.

12. Take advantage of packaged fresh salad greens for an instant easy salad.

13. Serve a festive vegetable-snacking platter at home or for parties. Include bell pepper rings and broccoli in addition to the usual veggie.

14. Add chopped tomatoes and other vegetables to burritos and tacos.

15. When eating out, ask yourself, How will I get a vegetable at this meal?

16. If eating a fast food meal try adding a baked potato, side salad, or a visit to the salad bar.

17. Chop a variety of different vegetables and toss them into your salad such as jícama and zucchini.

18. Add leftover vegetables to your favorite soup.

19. Stock your freezer with frozen vegetables so that you never have to do without.

20. Eat more vegetable-based meals in which they are an integral part of the dish such as stir-fries and pasta primavera.

✳ Sunburst Soup ✳

I'd never been a squash fan until this soup recipe. The creamy soup texture rather than a plain mound of vegetables has converted me. Yet this wonderful "cream" soup does not have a speck of fat. By the way fresh ginger is essential to the flavor; don't even think of substituting ground ginger. I love thick cream soups; if you prefer a thinner texture, feel free to add more chicken broth or thin with apple juice to the desired consistency.

THE SNEAK:

- The vegetable (butternut squash) is pureed.
- Strong spices (especially the fresh ginger) divert the taste buds.

NUTRITION SCORECARD (PER SERVING)		NOTABLE NUTRIENT (PER SERVING)		
Calories	139			
Fat (grams)	1.3		AMOUNT	% DAILY VALUE
% Fat calories	7			
Protein (grams)	6	Vitamin A (RE)	1914	191
Carbohydrates		Vitamin C (milligrams)	41	69
(grams)	30			
Cholesterol				
(milligrams)	1			

8	cups chunks of peeled butternut squash	1	teaspoon curry powder
4	cups chicken or vegetable broth	¼	teaspoon nutmeg
		¼	teaspoon cinnamon
2	tablespoons brown sugar	⅛	teaspoon ground cloves
1	tablespoon minced ginger (about 1-inch piece)		

Combine the squash, broth, brown sugar, minced ginger, curry powder, nutmeg, cinnamon, and cloves in a large pot or Dutch oven. Bring to a boil on high heat; reduce the heat to simmer and cover. Cook about 40 minutes or until the squash is tender.

Puree the squash mixture in a food processor or blender in small batches until smooth. (Or you can use a hand blender directly in the pot to puree the soup.) For a thinner consistency, add more chicken broth or add apple juice, if desired. Serve immediately.

Makes 6 servings (6 cups)

Is It a Fruit or Vegetable?

Culinary custom dictates which plant foods are considered vegetables or fruits, which often leads to some confusion. For example, these vegetables fit the botanical definition of fruit (the edible reproductive body of a seed plant): tomatoes, squash, avocado, and mature beans. The term vegetable is actually a generic botanical term for plant; therefore, you can say that every plant is a vegetable—now wouldn't that be more confusing?

Cancer Causes and Control 6:292–302, 1995

Cheddar Chowder

My family loves this soup and it makes for such a nourishing meal. I like my chowders on the thick side; if you wish a thinner consistency just add a little nonfat milk to suit your taste.

THE SNEAK:

- Finely grated carrots resemble little flecks of Cheddar cheese. (The easiest way to achieve this is to use a food processor.)

NUTRITION SCORECARD (PER SERVING)	
Calories	294
Fat (grams)	7.5
% Fat calories	22
Protein (grams)	24
Carbohydrates (grams)	35
Cholesterol (milligrams)	31

NOTABLE NUTRIENT (PER SERVING)	AMOUNT	% DAILY VALUE
Vitamin A (RE)	1824	182
Calcium (milligrams)	358	36

5	medium carrots, washed, ends cut off	2	(12-ounce) cans evaporated skim milk
3	celery stalks	⅓	cup cornstarch
1	small onion	½	teaspoon marjoram
3½	cups fat-free chicken broth	8	ounces (2 cups) shredded
1	large potato (¾ pound), peeled and diced (about 2 cups)		reduced-fat sharp Cheddar cheese

Using a food processor with a fitted blade, chop the carrots until they are very fine and resemble powdered Parmesan cheese, or use the smallest hole on a grater and shred the carrots. Transfer the carrots to a 4-quart saucepan. Using a food processor, chop the celery and onion and transfer to a pan.

Add the broth and diced potato to the pan. Bring to a boil and then reduce the heat. Cover and simmer about 10 minutes until the potatoes are tender. Using the back of a fork, slightly mash the potato against the side of the pan.

In a small cup, combine ¼ cup of the milk and the cornstarch and stir until smooth. Then stir the cornstarch mixture into the broth mixture. Add the remaining milk and marjoram. Cook and stir until thickened and bubbly. Cook and stir for 1 minute more. Slowly stir in the cheese. Remove from the heat and continue stirring until the cheese is melted.

Makes 6 main-course servings, about 1½ cups per serving

Vegetable Soup Counts!

Vegetable soups are the second largest source of provitamin A carotenoids in the American diet according to the data from the Second National Health and Nutrition Examination Survey (NHANES II).
Nutrition and Cancer 18:1–29, 1992

✖ Three-Pepper Confetti Pasta for Two ✖

This is one of my most requested recipes and one of my all-time favorite meals. It's so rich in flavor, super quick to prepare, and beautiful to serve. The advantage of using bell peppers is that they are a very forgiving vegetable—unlike temperamental veggies that wilt by the end of the week, peppers wait patiently to be eaten and enjoyed.
By the way this recipe can easily be doubled or tripled.
Quick tip: My favorite way to "dice" bell peppers is to use kitchen scissors. Remove the core and cut parallel vertical strips (it resembles a wig that can be thrown on a doll's head that's badly in need of a trim) horizontally!

THE SNEAK:

- Using vegetables (peppers) as a component of the meal rather than a side dish that prevents veggies from being forgotten or from falling between the nutritional cracks. This meal is loaded in vitamin C, thanks to the peppers, especially the yellow.

NUTRITION SCORECARD (PER SERVING)		NOTABLE NUTRIENT (PER SERVING)		
			AMOUNT	% DAILY VALUE
Calories	389			
Fat (grams)	9.9			
% Fat calories	23			
Protein (grams)	19	Vitamin A (RE)	305	31
Carbohydrates		Vitamin C (milligrams)	276	460
(grams)	56	Calcium (milligrams)	414	41
Cholesterol				
(milligrams)	22			

4   ounces dry angel hair pasta
3   cloves garlic, minced
1   red bell pepper, washed, seeded, and diced ¼ inch thick
1   yellow bell pepper, washed, seeded, and diced ¼ inch thick

1   green bell pepper, washed, seeded, and diced ¼ inch thick
2   ounces freshly grated Parmesan cheese (½ cup)

Cook the pasta according to the directions on the package. Drain and set aside.

Meanwhile, spray an unheated large skillet with olive oil nonstick spray. Add the garlic and cook until fragrant, about 30 seconds. Add the peppers. Cook and stir over medium-high heat for 3 to 5 minutes until slightly tender. (Take care not to overcook or the green pepper will turn a drab olive color.)

To serve: For maximum flavor I prefer to serve this meal as follows: Using two plates, arrange half of the cooked pasta between the two plates. On top of the pasta, add half of the pepper mixture and half of the Parmesan. Repeat using the remaining pasta, peppers, and cheese.

Makes 2 servings

Vegetables Protect Against Cancer

Of 194 studies examining the effects of diet and cancer prevention, vegetables in general and raw vegetables in particular had the most protective association.

Journal of the American Dietetic Association 96:1027–1039, 1996

❋ Home-Style Lasagna ❋

Unlike traditional vegetable lasagnas that scream "veggie," this dish subtly uses vegetables, discreetly added in itty-bitty pieces to the spaghetti sauce. As you can see the nutrition profile of one serving is quite impressive!

THE SNEAK:

- Incorporates finely grated carrots
- Adds chopped kale (looks like basil in the sauce)
- Adds diced red pepper

NUTRITION SCORECARD (PER SERVING)		NOTABLE NUTRIENT (PER SERVING)		
			AMOUNT	% DAILY VALUE
Calories	394			
Fat (grams)	10.6	Vitamin A (RE)	702	70
% Fat calories	24	Vitamin C (milligrams)	27	45
Protein (grams)	29	Calcium (milligrams)	530	53
Carbohydrates (grams)	47			
Cholesterol (milligrams)	35			

2	carrots, finely shredded	12	ounces lasagna noodles (12 noodles)	
1	cup loosely packed fresh kale, snipped like parsley	15	ounces fat-free ricotta cheese	
1	red bell pepper, diced	1	tablespoon all-purpose flour	
3	cloves garlic, minced	²/₃	cup shredded fresh Parmesan cheese, divided	
1	(26-ounce) jar low-fat spaghetti sauce	3	cups shredded part-skim mozzarella	
1	cup tomato sauce, divided			

Lightly spray an unheated large skillet with olive oil nonstick spray. Add the carrots, kale, pepper, and garlic. Cook and stir over medium heat for 5 minutes.

Stir in the spaghetti sauce and ²/₃ cup tomato sauce. Bring to a boil, then reduce the heat. Cover and simmer for 15 minutes.

Meanwhile, cook the lasagna noodles according to the directions on the package. Drain and set aside.

In a medium bowl, stir together the ricotta, flour, and ⅓ cup Parmesan cheese.

Preheat the oven to 350°F. To assemble, spread the remaining (⅓ cup) tomato sauce on the bottom of a 9- × 13-inch pan. Place four noodles in a single layer in the dish (they will slightly overlap). Spread ⅓ spaghetti sauce over the noodles. Add half of the ricotta cheese mixture by teaspoonful dollops. Sprinkle one third of the mozzarella cheese.

Repeat layers (⅓ noodles, ⅓ sauce, remaining ricotta, ⅓ mozzarella). On the final layer, use the remaining noodles, sauce, and mozzarella. Sprinkle on the remaining ⅓ cup Parmesan cheese. Bake for 40 to 45 minutes until golden and bubbly. Let stand for 10 minutes before cutting and serving.

Makes 8 generous servings

Carrot Power

Carrots in particular have shown to be protective against certain cancers, including breast, bladder, and mouth.
Journal of the American Dietetic Association 96:1027–1039, 1996

✳ Pesto Pasta Surprise ✳

A very simple recipe that requires no cooking except for boiling the noodles!

THE SNEAK:

• Broccoli is camouflaged under the familiar green color of pesto sauce.

NUTRITION SCORECARD (PER SERVING)		NOTABLE NUTRIENT (PER SERVING)		
			AMOUNT	% DAILY VALUE
Calories	395			
Fat (grams)	9.7			
% Fat calories	22			
Protein (grams)	20	Vitamin C (milligrams)	34	56
Carbohydrates (grams)	58			
Cholesterol (milligrams)	9			

12	ounces angel hair pasta or capellini	2	cups broccoli florets	
2	tablespoons pine nuts	4	teaspoons olive oil, divided	
½	cup fresh basil (leaves only)	¼	cup fat-free chicken broth	
5	cloves garlic, minced	⅔	cup freshly grated Parmesan cheese	
1	cup nonfat cottage cheese	1	tomato, diced	

Cook the pasta according to the directions on the package. Drain and set aside. If necessary, cover to keep warm.

Meanwhile, preheat the oven to 400°F. Place the pine nuts on a cookie sheet and bake 2 to 3 minutes until lightly golden. (Watch carefully to prevent burning.)

Transfer the pine nuts to a blender or food processor. Add the basil and garlic. Blend or process until finely chopped. Add the cottage cheese and blend until smooth. With the machine running, gradually add the broccoli and the olive oil. Then gradually add the chicken broth and Parmesan cheese.

In a large bowl toss the cooked pasta with the pesto and toss until well coated. Divide among five plates. Garnish with diced tomato.

Makes 5 servings

✳ Chicken Chili Verde ✳

It would be an understatement to say that my sister, Elaine, dislikes vegetables. So imagine my surprise when she shared this tasty recipe with me. Be forewarned this is a spicy dish, but ooh soo good.

THE SNEAK:

• The green vegetables look like chili.

NUTRITION SCORECARD (PER SERVING)		NOTABLE NUTRIENT (PER SERVING)		
			AMOUNT	% DAILY VALUE
Calories	149			
Fat (grams)	1.4			
% Fat calories	8			
Protein (grams)	22	Vitamin A (RE)	638	64
Carbohydrates (grams)	14	Folic acid (micrograms)	173	43
Cholesterol (milligrams)	45			

4 boneless, skinless chicken
    breasts
1 large onion, chopped
    (1½ cups)
2 cloves garlic
1 (1-pound) bunch spinach,
    washed, long stems
    removed, and finely chopped

½ cup cilantro, chopped
1 (7-ounce) can diced green
    chili
1 (10-ounce) package frozen
    french-cut green beans,
    thawed
1 cup mild green chili sauce

Spray an unheated 4-quart saucepan or Dutch oven with nonstick vegetable spray. Heat the skillet over medium heat. Add the chicken and cook about 4 minutes on each side until browned on the outside and the chicken is no longer pink on the inside. Remove the chicken from the pan. Using two forks, shred the chicken.

Using the same pan, add the onion and garlic. Cook and stir over medium heat until the onion is translucent, about 5 minutes. Stir in the shredded chicken, spinach, cilantro, green chili, thawed green beans, and chili sauce. Cover and simmer over low heat, stirring occasionally for 15 minutes.

Serving suggestions: roll into a burrito, stuff into a pita, or serve with brown rice.

Makes 6 servings (6 cups)

✺ Twice-Baked Potatoes ✺

This is a classic family favorite, yet when I incorporated a "mystery" vegetable into the mashed potatoes no one could even tell, including my daughter who claims not to like cauliflower. This is a great way to include a cruciferous vegetable especially if you haven't developed a liking for it!

THE SNEAK:

- Incorporating pureed cauliflower, which just happens to look like mashed potatoes and surprisingly has a neutral flavor in this form

NUTRITION SCORECARD (PER ONE POTATO—TWO HALVES)		NOTABLE NUTRIENT (PER SERVING)		
Calories	349			
Fat (grams)	5.6		AMOUNT	% DAILY VALUE
% Fat calories	14			
Protein (grams)	18	Vitamin C (milligrams)	148	247
Carbohydrates		Fiber (grams)	9	36
(grams)	61	Calcium (milligrams)	297	30
Cholesterol		Vitamin B$_6$ (milligrams)	1.1	55
(milligrams)	21			

4	medium potatoes, washed	¼	teaspoon black pepper
1½	pounds cauliflower, washed, green leaves removed	1	cup (4 ounces) finely shredded reduced-fat sharp Cheddar cheese
5	tablespoons nonfat milk, divided		paprika
¾	teaspoon salt		

Preheat the oven to 350°F. Using a fork, puncture the potatoes. Bake for 40 to 50 minutes until tender.

Meanwhile, cut the cauliflower into about eight pieces and steam until very tender. Transfer the cauliflower to a food processor or blender (in two batches if necessary). Add 2 tablespoons of the milk, salt, and pepper. Puree until smooth; the mixture will resemble mashed potatoes and make about 1 cup puree. Set aside.

Cut the potatoes in half lengthwise. Scoop out the pulp and place into a large mixing bowl, leaving thin shells. Using an electric mixer on lowest speed, beat the potato pulp and the remaining milk until blended. Add the pureed cauliflower mixture and beat until well mixed (do not overbeat). Stir in half of the shredded cheese.

Divide the mixture among the potato shells. Top with the remaining cheese and sprinkle with paprika. Return to the oven and bake until the cheese melts, about 5 minutes.

Makes 4 entree-size or 8 side-dish servings

✖ Garlicky Portobello Mushrooms ✖

These fabulous mushrooms are so incredible and rich in flavor. I get rave reviews every time I make them. They are quick and easy to prepare.

THE SNEAK:

• These Frisbee-sized mushrooms are not a subtle sneak, but I've had so many patients who were surprised that mushrooms "count" as vegetables that I included this favorite recipe to illustrate the point.

NUTRITION SCORECARD (PER SERVING)		NOTABLE NUTRIENT (PER SERVING)		
Calories	43			
Fat (grams)	1.7		AMOUNT	% DAILY VALUE
% Fat calories	29			
Protein (grams)	12	Fiber (grams)	3	12
Carbohydrates (grams)	5			
Cholesterol (milligrams)	1			

2	medium portobello mushrooms (5- to 6-inch diameter)	2	teaspoons chicken broth	
		3	cloves garlic, minced	
½	teaspoon olive oil	2	teaspoons freshly grated Parmesan cheese	

Preheat the oven to 400°F. Spray a baking sheet with nonstick spray. Gently rinse the mushrooms. Remove the stems (store and save for future use or discard). Pat the mushrooms dry with paper towels, especially the gills. Place the mushrooms, stem side up, on the prepared baking sheet.

Combine the olive oil, chicken broth, and garlic. Drizzle the garlic mixture over the mushrooms. Sprinkle with Parmesan cheese. Bake for 20 to 25 minutes until bubbly and the edges are somewhat shrunken.

VARIATION: Try topping the mushrooms with Italian Salsa (page 34).

Makes 2 servings

There's an Advantage to Cooked Vegetables

Cooking vegetables actually increases the availability of beta-carotene and some indoles (cancer-fighting phytochemicals) by degrading the cell wall in the plant, which helps to release these beneficial compounds.
Nutrition and Cancer 18:1–29, 1992

Pecan-Crusted Fluffy Sweet Potatoes

For several years when someone would say "pass the sweet potatoes," that's exactly what I did, passed them up every holiday season until I tasted a version of this recipe, now a family favorite. The whipped texture helped me cross over into becoming a sweet potato lover in any form. Canned or fresh sweet potatoes work equally well in this recipe.

THE SNEAK:

- Whipping the sweet potatoes

NUTRITION SCORECARD (PER SERVING)		NOTABLE NUTRIENT (PER SERVING)	AMOUNT	% DAILY VALUE
Calories	246			
Fat (grams)	6.7			
% Fat calories	24			
Protein (grams)	5	Vitamin A (RE)	1919	192
Carbohydrates (grams)	43	Vitamin E (milligrams)	4.7	47
Cholesterol (milligrams)	5			

WHIPPED POTATO

3½ cups cooked sweet potato pieces or 1 (40-ounce) can, drained
4 egg whites
2 tablespoons all-purpose flour

PECAN CRUST

⅓ cup packed brown sugar
2 tablespoons light butter
⅓ cup chopped pecans

Preheat the oven to 350°F. Spray a 9-inch pie plate with nonstick spray and set aside.

To make the whipped potatoes: Using a food processor or electric mixer, beat the sweet potatoes, egg whites, and flour just until smooth. Transfer the mixture to the prepared pie plate and bake for 15 minutes. Meanwhile, prepare the pecan crust.

To make the pecan crust: In a small microwavable bowl, add the brown sugar and light butter. Microwave on High for about 20 seconds until melted.

Carefully remove the sweet potatoes from the oven and top with the pecans. Drizzle the brown sugar mixture over the pecans. Return to the oven and bake an additional 15 minutes until golden and bubbly.

Makes 6 servings

Vitamin A Feast

Volunteers lunched daily on cooked kale and sweet potatoes, then washed it down with tomato juice. This special lunch provided ten times more than the typical U.S. diet for carotenoids (vitamin A). After just three weeks, the volunteers had a 33 percent increase in their immune response system.
USDA, AGS. Food and Nutrition Research Briefs, January 1997; page 1

Chinese Broccoli Slaw

Broccoli coleslaw is made up of primarily shredded hearts of broccoli and is sold nationwide (packaged) in the fresh produce section.

THE SNEAK:

- Using shredded hearts of broccoli

NUTRITION SCORECARD (PER SERVING)	
Calories	167
Fat (grams)	4.3
% Fat calories	23
Protein (grams)	3
Carbohydrates (grams)	29
Cholesterol (milligrams)	0

NOTABLE NUTRIENT (PER SERVING)	AMOUNT	% DAILY VALUE
Vitamin C (milligrams)	60	100

DRESSING

1/2 cup seasoned rice vinegar
1/3 cup fat-free chicken broth
1/3 cup pineapple juice
3 tablespoons sugar
2 tablespoons sesame oil
(dark brown)

SALAD

1 pound broccoli coleslaw or
6 cups finely shredded
cabbage
2 packages baked (fat-free)
ramen soup noodles, crum-
bled (discard the soup-
seasoning packet)
2/3 cup loosely packed snipped
fresh cilantro
1/2 cup snipped fresh chives

To make the dressing: In a small bowl whisk together the vinegar, broth, juice, sugar, and oil.

To make the salad: In a large bowl combine the broccoli coleslaw, *uncooked* noodles, cilantro, and chives. Add the dressing and toss until well coated. Cover and chill in the refrigerator for at least 1 hour until the noodles are soft.

Makes 8 servings (3/4 cup each)

✖ Italian Salsa ✖

This versatile salsa tastes great dipped with crusty bread, or better yet as topping over a pizza (see pizza recipe, page 151), or over pasta. The longer it sits in the refrigerator the better it tastes!

THE SNEAK:

• Adding chopped spinach with the basil (it looks identical)

NUTRITION SCORECARD (PER SERVING)		NOTABLE NUTRIENT (PER SERVING)		
			AMOUNT	% DAILY VALUE
Calories	40			
Fat (grams)	1.5			
% Fat calories	30			
Protein (grams)	1	Vitamin C (milligrams)	22	37
Carbohydrates (grams)	7			
Cholesterol (milligrams)	0			

4	cloves garlic, minced	¼	cup loosely packed fresh basil, snipped
1	teaspoon olive oil	⅛	teaspoon salt
1	pound Roma tomatoes (about 6 large), chopped		
⅓	cup loosely packed fresh spinach, snipped		

In a large microwavable bowl combine the garlic and olive oil. Microwave on High for 15 to 30 seconds, just until aromatic. Add the tomatoes, spinach, basil, and salt. Mix thoroughly to coat. Cover and chill until ready to serve.

Makes 4 servings (2 cups)

Carrot Cake Smoothie

Just as carrot cake does not taste like carrots, this smoothie does not taste like carrot juice. Try as I might I've always had difficulty drinking carrot juice straight, but in this beverage it is a pure pleasure. This drink allows me to enjoy the potent nutritional benefits of carrot juice.

THE SNEAK:

- Spiking the smoothie with carrot juice

NUTRITION SCORECARD (PER SERVING)		NOTABLE NUTRIENT (PER SERVING)	AMOUNT	% DAILY VALUE
Calories	219			
Fat (grams)	0			
% Fat calories	0			
Protein (grams)	5	Vitamin A (RE)	1052	105
Carbohydrates (grams)	49			
Cholesterol (milligrams)	0			

- 1/2 cup canned or fresh pineapple chunks (no juice)
- 1/3 cup carrot juice
- 3 scoops (1 1/2 cups) fat-free frozen vanilla yogurt
- 1/2 teaspoon coconut extract
- 1/8 teaspoon cinnamon
- 1/8 teaspoon nutmeg
- 1/2 to 1 cup ice

In a blender combine the pineapple chunks, carrot juice, frozen yogurt, coconut extract, cinnamon, and nutmeg. Blend until smooth. Add ice for the desired consistency.

Makes 2 servings (1-cup serving size)

✖ Pumpkin Pie Shake ✖

Such a delicious way to "eat" a vegetable year-round.

THE SNEAK:

• Canned pumpkin is the key ingredient that adds a lot of vitamin A.

NUTRITION SCORECARD (PER SERVING)		NOTABLE NUTRIENT (PER SERVING)		
Calories	249			
Fat (grams)	0		AMOUNT	% DAILY VALUE
% Fat calories	0			
Protein (grams)	7	Vitamin A (RE)	1801	180
Carbohydrates (grams)	55			
Cholesterol (milligrams)	0			

1	cup canned pumpkin	½	teaspoon pumpkin pie spice
1	cup nonfat milk	½	teaspoon rum extract
6	scoops (3 cups) fat-free frozen vanilla yogurt		

In a blender, combine the pumpkin, nonfat milk, frozen yogurt, pumpkin pie spice, and rum extract. Blend until smooth.

Makes 3 servings (generous 1 cup serving size)

Convenience—A Key to Eating Vegetables

Convenience and ease of preparation are the key factors that determined vegetable preferences among 150 adult men and women.
Journal of the American College of Nutrition 15(2):147–153, 1996

Try These Other Recipes with Vegetables

Artichoke Hummus	120
Chicken Salad with Creamy Lime–Cilantro Vinaigrette	203
Chili-Stuffed Potatoes	189
Chinese Beef Broccoli with Snow Peas	186
Curly Noodle Soup	98
Date Nut Bran Muffins	148
Denver Omelet	218
Fiesta Black Bean Salad	132
Fiesta Fajitas	179
Florentine Pasta Bundles	105
Garlic Mashed Potatoes	213
Lickety Split Pea Soup	126
Manhattan (Red) Clam Chowder	176
Old-fashioned Stuffing with Smoked Oysters	188
Onion Rings	214
Polenta with Fresh Corn	215
Pumpkin Custard with Gingersnap Crumble	109
Red Pepper Hummus with Roasted Garlic	121
Spaghetti with Sun-Dried Tomato Sauce	180
Spinach-Cheese Squares	71
Stir-fried Rice	160
Sweet and Sour Pork	211

CHAPTER TWO

Coming to Fruition

Fruits Make a Unique Difference

"I was dining out for dinner when it dawned on me that I had not eaten enough fruits for the day. After perusing the menu, I didn't see any fruit options—so I ordered a fresh peach margarita." When my client recalled this story, I knew that I had really gotten through to her the importance of fruit in the diet!

When fruits are lumped together with vegetables for healthful eating (as in the ubiquitous message of 5-A-Day for Health, sponsored by the National Cancer Institute), it's easy to forget that fruit in itself offers a unique nutrition advantage. Here are some examples:

• Several studies have shown that eating fruit in particular can help reduce the risk of various cancers.

• A chemical analysis of fruits (and juices) demonstrated that fruit contains special antioxidant powers that exceed what you would expect from vitamin C alone. In fact, fruits contain a group of naturally occurring antioxidants. One such group is called flavonoids. Flavonoids are associated with many healthful attributes, including antiinflammatory, antiallergic, and antihemorrhagic properties. One Dutch study that examined the health benefits of flavonoids found that a high consumption of dietary flavonoids was related to reduced deaths from heart disease and reduced incidence of a first fatal or nonfatal heart attack.

• A high fruit intake appears to improve lung function and may prove to be especially beneficial to asthmatics.

NUTRITIONAL GOLD MINE

Fruit also plays an important role in our diets with its bevy of nutrients, especially vitamins A, C, potassium, and fiber. Just one half of a cantaloupe provides 86 percent of your vitamin A needs a day, while supplying almost 200 percent of your vitamin C requirement. Take a look at the two charts, Fruits Super High in Vitamin A and Fruits Super High in Vitamin C, and you'll see how important fruits are for rounding out your diet.

JUICE: MORE IS NOT NECESSARILY BETTER

While the juicing trend brought a lot of attention to the health benefits of fruit, most of the beneficial parts of the fruit were being juiced right out, notably the fiber. Although juice certainly counts as a fruit serving, relying mainly on juice for your fruit servings can be a problem, especially for children.

• A study published in the journal *Pediatrics* (January 1997) found that preschool children who drank more than 12 ounces of juice a day were more than three times as likely to be overweight. This is equivalent to 1½ cups or 1½ packages of boxed juice.
• Excess fruit juice consumption has been reported as a contributing factor in some children with nonorganic failure to thrive (a condition in which children do not grow properly).
• Concomitant with the increase in fruit juice consumption there has been a decline in milk intake in children. This can be a problem because milk is the major source of calcium in the diet and at present only 50 percent of children aged one through five meet the Recommended Dietary Allowance for calcium.

What to do? It makes sense to limit juice consumption to one serving a day, which is about 6 ounces or ¾ cup a day (this is equal to one fruit serving in the Food Pyramid). When thirsty, consider other beverages such as water. Remember water is an essential nutrient. It's all too easy to guzzle juice calories when parched.

LIVING FRUITFULLY

• *How Much to Eat?*—aim for an absolute minimum of two servings each day, the more the better. It doesn't have to be two different fruits (although variety is always a great idea). Just doubling up on a fruit serving at breakfast will satisfy minimum fruit needs.

• *Fast Food and Restaurant Meals*—if you dine frequently on fast foods, it is a challenge to eat fruit. This is where drinking juice can be an asset, or be sure to include fruit as a snack or with another meal.

It's pretty easy to get fresh fruit on the breakfast menu at most restaurants, from berries to melon. At lunch and dinner, check out the menu for an entree-size fruit salad or a significant fruit garnish. Some restaurants have outstanding salad bars with a good selection of fresh fruit.

• *Good-Intentioned Fruit Eater*—according to a focus group survey conducted by the National Cancer Institute, the chief barrier to eating fruits was their perishable nature, and when out of season their expense and variable quality. If this reflects your obstacles to fruit consumption, keep these pointers in mind:

Keep a variety of fruits on hand, whether fresh, canned (juice pack, please), frozen, dried, or juice.

Develop the attitude that fruit is cost effective at any price. In the good old days when every penny counted (my bookcases were mere plywood boards propped up by cinderblock bricks), my husband and I had two prevailing spending rules: We would always have money for books and good food. That philosophy still remains. Ironically, I have friends who balk at buying expensive fruit, let's say raspberries, out of season at three dollars for a tiny basket, but don't think twice about spending the same amount for a cappuccino. So when fruit prices are high, just pretend that you're buying the Godiva of fruit for your body; remember it's an investment in your health.

There are many ways to try fruits or even sneak them into your diet.

Five Ways to Sneak Fruit into Meals

1. Puree a fruit and use it as a sauce, pudding, or smoothie. For example, see Mango Mousse, page 54.

2. Grate or chop a fruit into tiny almost undetectable bits. For example, see Cranberry-Orange Relish, page 48.

3. Suspend it—in gelatin that is. For example, see Tropical Orange Gelatin, page 56, in which orange juice is used as the liquid, studded with mandarin oranges and crushed pineapple.

4. Spice it up. Use strong sweet spices such as cinnamon and zest from lime, orange, or lemon. For example, see Breakfast Pudding, page 55.

5. Make fruit an integral part of a recipe rather than having it sit on the plate isolated. For example, see Strawberries and Cream Pie, page 49.

Fruits Super High in Vitamin A

These particular fruits are packed with vitamin A, providing at least 25 percent of what you need in a day.

Fruit	Vitamin A (RE)	%DV (percent Daily Value)
Apricot halves, dried, 10	253	25
Apricot nectar, 1 cup	330	33
Cantaloupe, 1/2 melon	861	86
Cantaloupe cubes, 1 cup	516	52
Honeydew cubes, 1 cup	307	31
Mango, 1	806	81
Papaya, 1 store ripened	127	13
Papaya, 1 sun ripened	602	60
Passionfruit juice (yellow), 1 cup	595	60
Persimmon, 1	364	36

Fruits Super High in Vitamin C

These particular fruits are packed with vitamin C, in many cases providing more than 60 milligrams or over 100 percent of what you need in one day.

Fruit	Vitamin C milligrams	%DV (percent Daily Value)
Blackberries, fresh, 1 cup	30	50
Cantaloupe, half	113	188
Cantaloupe cubes, 1 cup	68	113
Grapefruit, pink, half	47	78
Grapefruit, white, half	39	65
Grapefruit juice, 1 cup	83	138
Honeydew cubes, 1 cup	42	70
Kiwi, 1	75	125
Loganberries, 1 cup	52	87
Mango, 1	57	95
Orange, 1	70	117
Orange juice, 1 cup:		
from fresh	124	207
from frozen	97	162
from canned	86	143
Pineapple, 1 cup:		
fresh	24	40
canned, juice pack	24	40
Raspberries, 1 cup:		
fresh	31	52
frozen, thawed	41	68
Strawberries, 1 cup:		
fresh	85	142
frozen	61	102
Tangerine, 1	26	43
Tangerine juice, 1 cup	58	97

Canned Fruits: Sweetened versus Juice Pack

Your choice of canned fruit can have a significant calorie impact. Choose juice-packed fruits rather than heavy syrup-based fruits.

Canned Fruit	Calories
Fruit cocktail, 1 cup packed in:	
Juice	114
Light syrup	144
Heavy syrup	186
Peaches, 1 cup packed in:	
Juice	109
Light syrup	136
Heavy syrup	189
Pears, 2 halves, packed in:	
Juice	77
Light syrup	90
Heavy syrup	117

Twenty Ways to Increase Fruit in Your Diet

1. Buy fresh fruits in different stages of ripeness so they are ready to eat when you are.
2. Most of the health benefits of fruit are in the fiber and pulpy parts of fruit. Use primarily the whole fruit when making smoothies, a delicious way to add fruit into your diet.
3. Keep small packages of raisins and other dried fruits in a convenient place—briefcase, desk drawer, or glove compartment of your car.
4. Begin your day with two fruit servings such as berries or sliced banana with cereal and a glass of orange juice.
5. Keep convenient sources of fruit on hand when fresh isn't quite available. Include frozen fruit such as berries and canned fruit packed in its own juice.
6. Puree canned fruits such as apricots and use as sauce over low-fat ice cream or serve warm over pancakes for a real fruit syrup.
7. When traveling, don't forget about getting a fruit source with your meals, whether it's berries or melon with breakfast or orange juice with lunch.
8. Take advantage of freshly prepared fruit in the produce section of the grocery store such as melon balls and pineapple wedges.
9. Choose desserts that contain fruit such as a fresh fruit tart or berry-studded fruit sundae.
10. Take advantage of juice/smoothie bars. Opt for beverages that include whole fruit such as banana or strawberries.
11. Throw fruit into a gelatin for an appealing fruit snack.
12. When flying, request orange juice for your inflight beverage. If you don't like the canned taste, mix equal parts juice and club soda.
13. Add a fruit kebab to lunch by skewering some of your favorite fruits.
14. Start dinner with a fruit bowl appetizer. Fruit will easily get gobbled up with a hungry appetite.
15. Toss some dried fruits into your favorite muffin or cereal.
16. Try a fresh fruit topping on top of your favorite frozen yogurt.
17. Expand your fruit horizons; try a new fruit such as kiwi, mango, or star fruit or just a new variety of melon.
18. Be on the lookout for ways to add fruit to a recipe such as adding sliced oranges to a green salad.
19. Don't forget cooked fruits. If you have an oversupply of pears, peaches, or berries, make a fruit compote. Or bake the fruit with a sprinkle of cinnamon.
20. Entertain with fruit. Take a fruit platter or fruit basket to a party. Try a contemporary fruit fondue—hollow out a fat-free sponge cake and fill with a low-fat cream cheese dip. Serve with a platter of fresh fruit and skewers; strawberries work especially well.

Easy Kiwi Salad
❋ with Walnut Vinaigrette ❋

*The avocado tidbits combined with a hint of walnut oil in the dressing
enhance the flavor of this delicate fruit salad.*

THE SNEAK:

- Combining complementary fruit flavors with an outstanding dressing

NUTRITION SCORECARD (PER SERVING)		NOTABLE NUTRIENT (PER SERVING)		
			AMOUNT	% DAILY VALUE
Calories	256			
Fat (grams)	7.2			
% Fat calories	23			
Protein (grams)	3	Vitamin C (milligrams)	128	213
Carbohydrates		Fiber (grams)	10	40
(grams)	51			
Cholesterol				
(milligrams)	0			

SALAD

6 cups torn bibb lettuce or fresh
  baby spinach leaves
6 kiwi fruit, peeled and sliced
4 (10½-ounce) cans mandarin
  oranges, drained
1 avocado, peeled, pitted, and
  diced

WALNUT VINAIGRETTE DRESSING

1 tablespoon honey
2 teaspoons walnut oil
2 tablespoons fresh lime juice
¼ cup orange juice

To make the salad: Divide the lettuce among six salad plates. Add a layer
of kiwi slices, followed by a layer of mandarin oranges. Top with avocado
and drizzle with dressing.

To make the dressing: In a small bowl whisk together the honey and
walnut oil. Slowly whisk in the lime juice and orange juice.

Makes 6 servings

Ample Fruit Each Day Keeps Cancer Away

In twenty-eight of twenty-nine studies, fruits were found to be significantly protective against cancers of the oral cavity, larynx, esophagus, and rectum. And men who ate 2.5 servings of fruit per day showed a threefold protective effect against colon cancer compared with men who consumed one or fewer fruit servings per day.

Nutrition and Cancer 18:1–29, 1992

Cranberry-Orange Relish

I was never a fan of cranberries until an enthusiastic neighbor had me taste a version of this relish. When cranberries are in season, I make this at least once a week. Be sure to buy an extra bag or two of fresh cranberries in the fall and freeze them so that you can make this later in the year, too. The frozen cranberries come out remarkably well and you don't even need to thaw them to make this!

THE SNEAK:

- Cranberries are chopped into tiny bits.

NUTRITION SCORECARD (PER SERVING)	
Calories	155
Fat (grams)	0
% Fat calories	0
Protein (grams)	0.5
Carbohydrates (grams)	40
Cholesterol (milligrams)	0

NOTABLE NUTRIENT (PER SERVING)	AMOUNT	% DAILY VALUE
Fiber (grams)	4	17
Vitamin C (milligrams)	22	37

1 medium navel orange, unpeeled, washed
1/3 cup dried cranberries
1 (12-ounce) package fresh or frozen cranberries (do not thaw if frozen)
2/3 cup sugar

Cut the orange into eight wedges (with peel). Combine the sliced orange and dried cranberries in a food processor or blender. Pulse until coarsely chopped. Add the cranberries and sugar. Pulse until chopped evenly.

Makes 6 servings (¹/₂ cup each)

Appealing Orange Peel

The orange peel contains a biologically active compound, limonene, which has been shown to increase a detoxification enzyme which may help reduce cancer risk.

Journal of the American Dietetic Association 96:1027–1039, 1996

✳ Strawberries and Cream Pie ✳

This simple, gorgeous treat provides over 100 percent vitamin C needs for the day!

THE SNEAK:

- Over half of the strawberries are pureed and incorporated into the body of the pie. It's also a quick and easy way to use up berries that are on the verge of being overripe.

NUTRITION SCORECARD (PER SERVING)		NOTABLE NUTRIENT (PER SERVING)		
			AMOUNT	% DAILY VALUE
Calories	273			
Fat (grams)	4.6			
% Fat calories	16			
Protein (grams)	13	Protein (grams)	13	29
Carbohydrates		Fiber (grams)	5	20
(grams)	44	Vitamin C (milligrams)	64	106
Cholesterol				
(milligrams)	4			

⅓ cup nonfat milk
2 packets gelatin
1 (16-ounce) container nonfat cottage cheese
⅓ cup sugar
4½ cups strawberries, washed and hulled, divided

1 ready-made low-fat graham cracker crust
1 tablespoon seedless strawberry jam

Add the milk to a small saucepan. Sprinkle the gelatin over the milk and let stand 1 minute until the liquid is completely absorbed. (This mixture will liquefy once you begin cooking.) Cook and stir over medium heat until dissolved, 2 to 3 minutes; do not boil. Set aside.

In a food processor or blender, combine the cottage cheese and sugar. Puree until smooth and creamy (resembling sour cream). Add 2½ cups strawberries to the food processor or blender and puree until smooth. Gradually mix in the gelatin mixture. Pour the strawberry cottage cheese mixture into the graham cracker crust. Cover and chill until slightly set, about 30 minutes.

Meanwhile, cut the remaining strawberries in half. Arrange the strawberries decoratively over the filled pie crust. Place the jam in a small microwavable cup and microwave about 15 seconds until melted. Glaze the strawberries with the melted jam. Return the pie to the refrigerator and chill until set, about 2 hours.

Makes 6 servings

Strawberries for Brainpower

The antioxidant properties in strawberries may help brainpower if rat studies by USDA and University of Denver scientists are any indication. Rats were exposed to high levels of oxygen for two days to mimic the aging process that occurs in human brains. The rats that ate strawberry extracts as part of their diets fared dramatically better on a battery of tests that reflect memory and nerve cell function.
USDA, AGS. *Food and Nutrition Research Briefs,* April 2, 1997

✖ Fresh Blueberry Bavarian ✖

Here's another winning example of how fruit can be incorporated into a mouth-watering dessert.

THE SNEAK:

- The blueberry topping uses primarily fresh, uncooked fruit, which enhances the nutrient retention.

NUTRITION SCORECARD (PER SERVING)		NOTABLE NUTRIENT (PER SERVING)		
Calories	230			
Fat (grams)	5		AMOUNT	% DAILY VALUE
% Fat calories	21			
Protein (grams)	9	Fiber (grams)	3	12
Carbohydrates (grams)	37	Vitamin C (milligrams)	17	28
Cholesterol (milligrams)	23			

BAVARIAN

¾ cup nonfat milk

1 packet (2 teaspoons) unflavored gelatin

⅓ cup sugar

8 ounces fat-free cream cheese, softened at room temperature

3 ounces regular cream cheese, softened at room temperature

1 teaspoon almond extract

FRESH BLUEBERRY TOPPING

4 cups fresh blueberries, divided

3 tablespoons sugar

1 teaspoon cornstarch

¼ teaspoon cinnamon

¼ teaspoon nutmeg

3 tablespoons fresh lemon juice

To make the Bavarian: Add the milk to a medium saucepan. Sprinkle the gelatin over the milk and let stand while preparing the blueberry topping, at least 1 minute. Add the sugar to the gelatin mixture. Cook and stir over medium heat until the gelatin is dissolved (do not boil), about 2 to 3 minutes. Remove from the heat.

In a large bowl beat the cream cheeses with an electric mixer on medium speed until smooth. While beating, drizzle in the gelatin mixture and almond extract. Pour the cream cheese mixture into six 8-ounce ramekins or individual soufflé dishes. Chill while making the blueberry topping.

To make the fresh blueberry topping: Finely chop ⅔ cup blueberries in a food processor or blender. Transfer to a medium saucepan. Mix together the sugar, cornstarch, cinnamon, and nutmeg and add to the mixture the chopped blueberries. Stir in the lemon juice. Cook and stir over medium heat until the mixture thickens and boils. Remove from the heat. Add the remaining 3⅓ cups blueberries and toss to coat. Spoon the mixture on top of the individual Bavarians. Cover and chill until set, about 2 hours.

Makes 6 servings

A Berry Special Fruit

Of forty fruits and vegetables tested, blueberries by far had the highest antioxidant score. In fact only two thirds of a cup of berries had the same antioxidant power as 1270 milligrams of vitamin C—that's equivalent to 21 times the RDA level of vitamin C.
  USDA, AGS. Food and Nutrition Research Briefs, January 2, 1997

According to the results of the Minnesota Adolescent Health Survey, frequent dieting was associated with inadequate fruit intake of 36,284 students in grades seven to twelve.
  Preventive Medicine 25(Sept./Oct.):497–505, 1996

❈ Warm Blackberry Crustless Pie ❈

Fresh blackberries have a short season, but this treat can be eaten year-round thanks to the convenience of frozen berries. This dessert is a cross between a crustless pie and a cobbler with a built-in sour cream topping. It was such a hit with my family that they begged me not to ration it off to the neighborhood taste-testers!

THE SNEAK:

- This is a nice example of using fruit as a component in dessert—and who doesn't love dessert!

NUTRITION SCORECARD (PER SERVING)		NOTABLE NUTRIENT (PER SERVING)		
Calories	217			
Fat (grams)	0.5		AMOUNT	% DAILY VALUE
% Fat calories	2			
Protein (grams)	5	Fiber (grams)	4	16
Carbohydrates (grams)	49			
Cholesterol (milligrams)	trace			

1	(1-pound bag) frozen blackberries (do not thaw)
3	tablespoons dry bread crumbs
2	tablespoons sugar, plus ¾ cup sugar
1	teaspoon cinnamon
2	tablespoons quick-cooking tapioca
1	cup fat-free sour cream
¼	cup all-purpose flour

Preheat the oven to 375°F. Arrange the blackberries evenly on a 9-inch pie plate. In a small cup combine the bread crumbs, 2 tablespoons sugar, and cinnamon. Sprinkle half of the bread-crumb mixture and the tapioca over the berries.

In a small bowl mix together the sour cream, ¾ cup sugar, and flour. Pour this mixture evenly over the bread-crumb layer. Sprinkle the remaining bread-crumb mixture on top of the sour-cream mixture. Bake for 35 minutes until bubbly and golden. Serve warm in six dessert bowls.

Makes 6 servings

Mango Mousse
✖ with Raspberry Speckles ✖

This mousse is so incredibly good—by far one of my favorite ways to enjoy fruit! Even my daughter who does not like mangoes loved this and wanted to be sure that I passed on her surprised delight to you. Note: You may be able to reduce the amount of sugar, depending upon the ripeness of the mango.

THE SNEAK:

• Mango is pureed and provides a lovely background flavor for this mousse.

NUTRITION SCORECARD (PER SERVING)		NOTABLE NUTRIENT (PER SERVING)		
Calories	188			
Fat (grams)	0.6		AMOUNT	% DAILY VALUE
% Fat calories	3			
Protein (grams)	3	Vitamin A (RE)	365	36
Carbohydrates		Vitamin C (milligrams)	35	58
(grams)	43	Fiber (grams)	6	24
Cholesterol				
(milligrams)	3			

¾ cup nonfat milk, divided
1 packet (2 teaspoons) gelatin
1 (12-ounce) mango, peeled, cut into chunks, or 1½ cups frozen mango, thawed
½ cup fat-free sour cream

⅓ cup sugar
1 teaspoon rum extract
1 (6-ounce) container fresh raspberries, washed and drained

In a small saucepan add ¼ cup of the milk and sprinkle the gelatin over. Let stand for 5 minutes (the mixture will resemble cooked cream of wheat). Cook and stir over medium-low heat until the gelatin dissolves, about 5 minutes (do not boil). Remove from the heat and let cool while preparing the mango puree.

In a blender, combine the mango, sour cream, sugar, rum extract, and remaining milk. Blend on high speed until smooth. Add the gelatin mixture and blend again. Pour into four 6-ounce custard cups. Divide the berries among the cups. Cover with plastic and chill until firm, about 1 hour or overnight.

Makes 4 servings

Fresh Fruit Improves Breathing

Eating fresh fruit may make it easier to breathe for children, especially for those with asthma. Researchers from London examined the diets of 2650 children aged eight to eleven. Children with the highest fruit intake had the best lung function as measured by a procedure called forced expiratory volume. Conversely, children who never ate any fresh fruit had a significantly lower lung function compared to those who ate at least one fresh fruit serving a day.
Thorax 52(July):628–633, 1997

✖ Breakfast Pudding ✖

This is one of my favorite breakfasts—one batch lasts most of the week.

THE SNEAK:

- Orange juice and cinnamon infuse the prunes with an appealing flavor, while pureeing this fiber-rich fruit provides a mellow texture.

NUTRITION SCORECARD (PER SERVING)		NOTABLE NUTRIENT (PER SERVING)		
Calories	196			
Fat (grams)	<0.5		AMOUNT	% DAILY VALUE
% Fat calories	2			
Protein (grams)	5	Fiber (grams)	6	24
Carbohydrates		Vitamin C (milligrams)	33	55
(grams)	52			
Cholesterol				
(milligrams)	0			

1	(12-ounce) package pitted prunes (about 2 cups)	1	teaspoon cinnamon
1½	cups orange juice	¼	teaspoon nutmeg
2	(8-ounce) containers nonfat vanilla yogurt		

Combine the prunes and orange juice in a medium saucepan and bring to a boil over medium heat. Remove from the heat, cover, and set aside for 30 minutes or longer.

Puree the prunes with all of the orange juice in two batches in a food processor or blender. Gently fold in the vanilla yogurt until blended. Stir in the cinnamon and nutmeg. Transfer to six 6-ounce custard cups. Cover and refrigerate at least 2 hours or overnight.

Makes 6 servings (³/₄ cup each)

✖ Tropical Orange Gelatin ✖

I like to eat this for a refreshing breakfast or snack. The orange juice concentrate not only adds a rich source of vitamin C but it sets the gelatin quicker.

THE SNEAK:

- Orange juice is used for the main liquid.
- Carrot juice is added for color, sweetness, and vitamin A.

NUTRITION SCORECARD (PER SERVING)		NOTABLE NUTRIENT (PER SERVING)		
Calories	175			
Fat (grams)	0		AMOUNT	% DAILY VALUE
% Fat calories	0			
Protein (grams)	5	Vitamin A (RE)	569	57
Carbohydrates		Vitamin C (milligrams)	75	125
(grams)	41			
Cholesterol				
(milligrams)	0			

4	packets plain gelatin	1	(20-ounce can) crushed
2 1/2	cups water, divided		pineapple, juice-packed,
2/3	cup carrot juice		(do not drain)
1	(12-ounce) can orange juice	2	(10 1/2-ounce can) mandarin
	concentrate (do not thaw)		oranges, drained

In a large saucepan sprinkle the gelatin over 1½ cups water. On medium heat, cook and stir the gelatin until dissolved and translucent, about 5 minutes. In a large bowl combine the gelatin mixture, remaining water, carrot juice, and orange juice concentrate. Add the crushed pineapple with juice and the mandarin oranges to the remaining orange juice gelatin mixture. Divide the gelatin mixture among 8 dessert cups. Cover and chill until set, about 1 hour.

QUICK METHOD: Follow the above directions, except use a bundt pan instead of the dessert cups. Be sure to chill for at least 2 hours before unmolding.

Makes 8 servings

✖ Purple Cow sMOOthie ✖

The berries and juice create a delightful purple color—kids love the name and taste of this drink.

THE SNEAK:

• Pureeing berries into a shake

NUTRITION SCORECARD (PER SERVING)		NOTABLE NUTRIENT (PER SERVING)		
Calories	296			
Fat (grams)	0.6		AMOUNT	% DAILY VALUE
% Fat calories	2			
Protein (grams)	6	Fiber (grams)	4	17
Carbohydrates		Vitamin C (milligrams)	25	42
(grams)	68			
Cholesterol				
(milligrams)	0			

| 1 | cup of frozen mixed berries (blueberries, blackberries, strawberries, raspberries) | 1½ | scoops (¾ cup) nonfat frozen yogurt |
| 2/3 | cup berry juice (blackberry, boysenberry, black currant) | | |

Add the berries and juice to a blender and puree until smooth. Add the frozen yogurt and blend until the desired consistency.

Makes 1 (about 1¹/₄ cups) serving

Fruit juice accounts for 50 percent of all fruit servings consumed by children aged two to eighteen.
Journal of the American College of Nutrition 15(Oct.):4s–11s, 1996

✖ Lime-Kiwi Quencher ✖

This lip-puckering, daquirilike slush provides over twice your vitamin C needs for the day. For a fizzier variation, try substituting club soda for the pineapple juice.

THE SNEAK:

- Kiwis blend right into the background with their green color and they boost the vitamin C content tremendously.

NUTRITION SCORECARD (PER SERVING)		NOTABLE NUTRIENT (PER SERVING)		
Calories	240			
Fat (grams)	0.6			
% Fat calories	2		AMOUNT	% DAILY VALUE
Protein (grams)	1	Fiber (grams)	4	16
Carbohydrates		Vitamin C (milligrams)	127	212
(grams)	62			
Cholesterol				
(milligrams)	0			

3	kiwi, peeled and sliced	1	finely grated lime peel (save the
½	cup pineapple juice		remaining lime for garnish)
½	cup frozen limeade concentrate, partially thawed	1½	to 2 cups ice cubes

In a blender combine the kiwi, pineapple juice, limeade, and lime peel. Cover and blend until smooth. With the blender running, add the ice cubes, one at a time, through the opening in the lid. Blend until slushy and at the desired consistency. Pour into large glasses. Garnish with lime slices and serve immediately.

Makes 2 (12-ounce) servings

Apples Protective Against Ulcers

Fruits and vegetables, especially those high in fiber and vitamin A, may protect against ulcers. In a six-year study of more than forty-seven thousand men, researchers found that those who ate seven or more servings of fruits and vegetables daily had about a 30 percent lower risk in developing an ulcer compared to those who ate less than three servings a day. One fruit that stood out as particularly protective in this study was apples.
American Journal of Epidemiology 145(Jan 1):42–50, 1997

✖ Cantaloupe Cooler ✖

Partially freezing the cantaloupe gives this beverage a colder, refreshing edge. If you don't want to wait for the freezing effect, just plop in a couple of ice cubes while blending.

THE SNEAK:

• Cantaloupe is pureed into a refreshing shake.

NUTRITION SCORECARD (PER SERVING)		NOTABLE NUTRIENT (PER SERVING)		
			AMOUNT	% DAILY VALUE
Calories	295			
Fat (grams)	<0.5			
% Fat calories	1			
Protein (grams)	4	Vitamin A (RE)	516	52
Carbohydrates		Vitamin C (milligrams)	68	113
(grams)	66			
Cholesterol				
(milligrams)	0			

1   cup cantaloupe chunks (about ⅓ melon), partially frozen (at least 1 to 2 hours)

2   tablespoons white grape juice
2   scoops (1 cup) fat-free frozen vanilla yogurt

Add the cantaloupe and juice to a blender and puree until smooth. Add the frozen yogurt and blend until the desired consistency.

Makes 1 serving (about 1 cup)

Grapes and Resveratrol

Researchers have identified a cancer-fighting compound in grapes called resveratrol. This mighty phytochemical prevents cell-damaging mutations, blocks the development of tumors, and inhibits the growth and spread of cancer in mice.

Science 275(January 10):218–229, 1997

✖ Paradise Shake ✖

One sip of this refreshing shake and you'll be transported to an island paradise.

THE SNEAK:

• A whole papaya is pureed and blended into the shake.

NUTRITION SCORECARD (PER SERVING)		NOTABLE NUTRIENT (PER SERVING)		
Calories	260			
Fat (grams)	0		AMOUNT	% DAILY VALUE
% Fat calories	0			
Protein (grams)	7	Fiber (grams)	3	12
Carbohydrates		Vitamin A (RE)	337	34
(grams)	59	Vitamin C (milligrams)	119	198
Cholesterol				
(milligrams)	1			

1	(12-ounce) papaya, peeled, seeded, and cut into chunks	⅓	cup nonfat milk
¼	cup fresh lime juice	1	teaspoon coconut extract
¼	cup orange juice	1½	cups frozen vanilla yogurt

Add the papaya to a blender and puree until smooth. Add the lime juice, orange juice, milk, and coconut extract and blend. Add the frozen yogurt and blend until the desired consistency.

Makes 2 servings (about 1 cup each)

Guava Fruit Lowers Blood Pressure

Volunteers who added guava fruit to their diet had a substantial decrease in blood pressure and cholesterol levels compared to a group of patients who had an identical diet without guava.
Journal of Human Hypertension 7(Feb. 3):33–38, 1993

Try These Other Recipes with Fruit

CHAPTER THREE

Calcium Quota

Calcium: An Important Mineral for Men and Women

As a health professional, I've certainly been familiar with the bone-robbing disease, osteoporosis. But not until my grandmother had this terrible condition did I truly understand the impact of this *preventable* disease. She suffered fracture after fracture, and I watched her lose nearly six inches (no exaggeration) while her quality of life deteriorated.

One problem with osteoporosis is that it is truly a silent disease until a fracture occurs late in life. When you are not getting enough calcium—the body just turns to its built-in Fort Knox of calcium, bone. You do not feel your bones silently slipping away, hollowing out over the years. Unfortunately, Americans are building a huge deficit when it comes to their bone health. The typical American gets only 600 milligrams of calcium each day, which is a far cry from the recommended adult levels of 1000 to 1500 milligrams.

One in 2 women over the age of fifty suffers from fractures due to osteoporosis. Researchers estimate that 28 million Americans suffer from or are at high risk of developing osteoporosis and predict that the prevalence could rise to 41 million by the year 2015 unless steps are taken to prevent the disease. And don't be fooled into thinking that this is just a disease that affects women. *Men are also at risk* and suffer 20 to 25 percent of all hip fractures in the United States. While there is less research on men, the studies that do exist show that an inadequate calcium intake in men is associated with reduced bone mass and increased fracture risk.

While there are many factors that contribute to developing osteoporosis (including physical activity and family history), we will focus primarily on the role of calcium.

CALCIUM MAKES A DIFFERENCE AT ANY STAGE OF LIFE

It's important to remember that the human skeleton, bone, is active, living tissue. It is constantly taking in and releasing calcium. It is the balance of this give-and-take of calcium that affects peak bone mass, or optimal density of bone. Bone mass peaks at twenty-five to thirty years of age for women and thirty to thirty-five for men. So those of you coming to this age range want to do everything possible to ensure maximum bone density. (For those of you beyond these years, don't worry, it's not all over.) Storing calcium to make dense (healthy) bones over the years is similar to establishing a nest egg or savings account whose dividends you plan to live off at retirement. The more you save, the better your future. But withdraw too much or fail to contribute, and you may wind up broke (pun intended).

Optimal calcium intake in childhood and young adulthood is critical to achieving optimal bone mass. Research at the National Institute of Child Health and Human Development (NICHD) has found that an extra 350 milligrams of calcium per day (that's equivalent to one cup of milk or yogurt) can increase bone density in adolescent girls by 14 percent. At first glance these numbers may not be striking, but consider that for every 5 percent increase in bone density, the risk of bone fractures decreases by 40 percent. The problem, however, is that most teens fail miserably in getting enough calcium in their diet during these important bone-building years.

Once peak adult bone mass is reached, the bone metabolism is in balance. The bone is no longer building its density, and it is not being hollowed out.

During menopausal years bone loss accelerates and continues, in large part due to the absence of estrogen. Getting enough calcium is very important during these years to limit the loss of bone. Studies on average show that individuals who receive a combination of estrogen and calcium have a threefold increase in bone mass compared to those who receive estrogen alone.

In men and women sixty-five years of age, age-related bone loss continues, but can actually worsen because calcium absorption (the amount of calcium that you eat that actually gets inside the body) is reduced. The NIH Consensus Panel on Optimal Calcium concluded that the prevailing calcium intakes in this group are insufficient to prevent calcium-related erosion of bones.

BEYOND BONES—CALCIUM'S OTHER IMPORTANT ROLES

As if healthy bones are not reason enough to make sure you get enough calcium, there are many promising studies that show calcium does a lot more for health. Calcium may:

• Reduce colon cancer risk. It appears that calcium protects the colon by forming what's known as a calcium soap. Calcium soaps neutralize the irritating effect of bile acids and fatty acids in the bowel.
• Prevent a medical condition during pregnancy called preeclampsia, a serious problem in which high blood pressure, fluid retention, and protein in the urine develop in women during the second half of pregnancy.
• Decrease risk for kidney stones. This is true only of calcium from food sources, though, not calcium supplements. Ironically, calcium supplements may raise kidney stone risk.

Does it matter where you get your calcium from? Most authorities, including the NIH Consensus Panel on Optimal Calcium Intake, recommend food first. The most apparent choices come from dairy foods (low fat, of course), because they provide a rich source of calcium (see the Calcium-Rich Foods chart, page 68). If, however, you are vegetarian and choose not to eat dairy, you need to be sure that you are getting some high-calcium food sources (see the Nondairy Calcium-Rich Foods chart, page 69).

Lactose Intolerance. If you have an inability to digest the milk sugar, lactose, there are plenty of choices available from lactose-free milk products to lactase tablets, which break down the milk sugar in the food before you eat. You may even be able to tolerate some lactose. Research from Kent State and Purdue universities, reported in *Environmental Nutrition,* found that people who are lactose intolerant can adapt to large doses of lactose, thanks to a little help from friendly bacteria in the large intestine, called Bifidobacteria. The bacteria adapts to the constant supply of lactose at meals and learns to break the lactose down. The key is drinking ½ cup to 1 cup of milk with meals on a regular basis.

Using the Food Label. You can use the food label to your advantage by reading the Nutrition Facts panel. Look for the "percent Daily Value" (%DV) for calcium. It's a quick guide that lets you know how a particular food measures up in the calcium department. The higher the number the better. Fortunately, there are some legal definitions:
- 20 percent DV or more: the food is high in calcium
- 10 to 19 percent DV: the food contains a good source of calcium

If a food has 10 percent DV calcium or more added, it can state on the label "calcium enriched," "calcium fortified," or "more calcium."

Supplements. If you have trouble getting adequate calcium from your diet you should consider a calcium supplement. Check out the Calcium Supplement Tips below.

Calcium Supplement Tips

While the preferred approach to getting optimal calcium is through food, the next best is to consider a supplement. Keep these tips in mind:

- Calcium is best absorbed at doses of 500 milligrams or less.
- For most healthy people, the best time to take the supplement is between meals for better calcium absorption.
- Don't rely on a general multivitamin/multimineral supplement for calcium; the levels are generally very low.
- If you are taking iron supplements, take them at a different time than the calcium pills. Calcium supplements interfere with iron absorption.
- Do not exceed 2000 milligrams of supplemental calcium.

Optimal Calcium Intake. NIH Consensus Statement 1994 June 6–8; 12(4):1–31

BONING UP

• *How Much to Eat?*—aim for an absolute minimum of three calcium-rich servings each day. It doesn't have to be dairy products, but they are the richest source of calcium. Keep these recommended calcium levels from the Institute of Medicine's Food and Nutrition Board in mind:

Age (Male and Female)	Calcium (milligrams/day)
4–8 years	800
9–18	1300
19–50	1000
51 +	1200
PREGNANCY	
<19	1300
19–50	1000
BREASTFEEDING	
<19	1300
19–50	1000

• *If You Are Vegetarian and Dairy-Free*—don't make the mistake of eliminating dairy and not replacing it with calcium-rich foods such as extra-firm tofu (made with calcium sulfate), dark leafy greens, and fortified calcium products.

• *Good-Intentioned Milk Drinker*—according to a USDA survey comparing 1994 daily beverages with those in the late 1970s, many people switched from milk to other drinks. The number one beverage? Soda. Replacing milk with nondairy drinks like soda or tea is a habit that shortchanges your calcium. Drinking low-fat or nonfat milk is one of the easiest ways to get calcium; try making it a habit for at least one meal such as breakfast or dinner.

• *Milk Resisters*—perhaps you dislike drinking milk (actually you can count me in that category) but don't mind "eating" milk in foods such as macaroni and cheese, or pudding. Or perhaps it's an issue of disliking milk "straight" as a beverage; this is where such other beverages as lattè or hot chocolate can provide an inviting source of calcium.

There are many ways to sneak calcium into your diet. Since low-fat dairy products are the easiest way to get calcium in the diet, the recipes in this chapter are dairy-based.

Calcium-Rich Foods

Food	Calcium (milligrams)	% DV (percent Daily Value)	Calories
Buttermilk, 1 cup	285	29	99
Cheese, 1 ounce:			
Cheddar	204	20	114
Cheddar, reduced fat	253	25	81
Monterey Jack	211	21	106
Monterey Jack, reduced fat	253	25	81
Mozzarella, reduced fat	207	21	80
Parmesan	389	39	129
Romano	301	30	110
Swiss	272	27	107
Swiss, reduced fat	272	27	51
Milk, 1 cup:			
skim/nonfat	302	30	86
1% low fat	300	30	102
2% low fat	297	30	121
Milk, evaporated skim (fat-free), ½ cup	369	37	100
Milk, instant nonfat dry, ¼ cup	209	21	61
Ricotta cheese, part skim, ½ cup	334	33	170
Yogurt, nonfat, 1 cup	452	45	127
Yogurt, frozen, 1 cup	206	21	228

Nondairy Calcium-Rich Foods

Food	Calcium (milligrams)	% DV (Daily Value)	Calories
Almonds, whole, 2 ounces	151	15	334
Amaranth grain, ½ cup	149	15	364
Corn tortillas, 3 (6-inch each)	126	13	195
Dandelion greens, cooked, 1 cup	147	15	35
Figs, dried, 6 each	161	16	286
Mustard greens, cooked, 1 cup	152	15	29
Orange juice, calcium fortified, 1 cup	300–350	30–35	110
Sardines, w/bone, 8	365	37	199
Sesame seeds, 2 tablespoons	176	18	103
Soybeans, boiled	175	18	298
Tofu, firm, ½ cup	258	26	181
Turnip greens, cooked, 1 cup	250	25	49

Twenty Ways to Increase Calcium in Your Diet

1. When preparing oatmeal or other hot cereals, make it with low-fat milk.
2. Spread ricotta cheese on raisin toast for a midmorning snack.
3. Try calcium-fortified foods such as orange juice.
4. Add milk instead of nondairy creamer to your coffee.
5. Buy extra-firm tofu rather than softer varieties—it has more calcium.
6. Prepare cream soups with evaporated skim milk instead of cream. Ounce for ounce, evaporated skim milk has nearly five times the amount of calcium compared to cream.
7. Add a slice of low-fat cheese to your favorite sandwich.
8. Have a sweet tooth? Try puddings or low-fat frozen yogurt for a satisfying calcium kick.
9. Try having a bowl of cold cereal with nonfat milk for a snack.
10. Make your own hot chocolate; many instant varieties don't have the calcium. Simply combine a few teaspoons of chocolate syrup with milk and heat in the microwave.
11. Sprinkle low-fat cheese on your favorite vegetables, chili, or baked potato.
12. Use nonfat plain yogurt instead of sour cream for making your favorite dip mix. Ounce for ounce, yogurt has nearly twice the amount of calcium than sour cream.
13. Order low-fat milk for your beverage at a fast food restaurant. Be sure to request milk instead of soda for kiddy meals—it's no extra charge.
14. Make a low-fat quesadilla. Top a whole wheat flour tortilla with low-fat Cheddar or Jack cheese. Add salsa if desired and microwave until melted.
15. For a satisfying snack, choose yogurt; it's one of the highest sources of calcium in the diet. But to get your calcium's worth out of yogurt, be sure to purchase the eight-ounce size rather than the smaller container.
16. When in the mood for Italian cuisine, choose foods with ricotta (preferably low fat or fat free) such as manicotti, lasagna, or ravioli. Ricotta has eight times the calcium of cottage cheese.
17. Switch to fat-free cream cheese instead of regular. Fat-free cream cheese has milk solids added to it, which boosts the calcium to nearly four times the amount found in regular cream cheese.
18. Add some pizza pizzazz to your meals. Not only is it a great source of calcium but it's an opportunity to add vegetable toppings.
19. Add nonfat dried powdered milk to recipes such as soups, casseroles, and cookie doughs.
20. Keep some low-fat snack cheeses on hand such as string cheese.

❈ Spinach-Cheese Squares ❈

This crustless quiche gives a little kick to the taste buds with the diced green chilies. It's a hit with my family and so easy to prepare.

THE SNEAK:

- The built-in cheese adds a rich calcium source.
- Spinach also makes a significant nondairy calcium contribution.

NUTRITION SCORECARD (PER SERVING)		NOTABLE NUTRIENT (PER SERVING)		
Calories	210			
Fat (grams)	6.9			
% Fat calories	32		AMOUNT	% DAILY VALUE
Protein (grams)	23	Vitamin A (RE)	58	58
Carbohydrates		Calcium (milligrams)	396	40
(grams)	13			
Cholesterol				
(milligrams)	59			

6   egg whites
1   whole egg
⅓   cup all-purpose flour
1   teaspoon dry mustard powder
½   teaspoon baking powder
1   (10-ounce) package frozen chopped spinach, thawed and well drained

1   (4-ounce) can diced green chilies
1   cup nonfat cottage cheese
1   cup shredded reduced-fat sharp Cheddar cheese
1   cup shredded reduced-fat Swiss cheese

Preheat the oven to 350°F. Spray a 10- × 10-inch baking pan with non-stick vegetable spray.

In a large bowl use an electric mixer on low to beat the egg whites and whole egg. Mix in the flour, dry mustard, and baking powder. Do not overmix or the final product will be tough. Beat in the spinach, green chilies, cottage cheese, Cheddar cheese, and Swiss cheese.

Pour the mixture into the prepared pan. Bake for 45 to 50 minutes until golden brown and the center is set. Remove from the oven and let stand for 15 minutes. Cut into six squares and serve.

Makes 6 servings

❊ Cheesy Stuffed Shells ❊

This is a meal you'll want to make over and over again. It's hard to believe that just one serving provides nearly two thirds of the recommended calcium level.

THE SNEAK:

• Nonfat dried milk is added to the ricotta cheese filling.

NUTRITION SCORECARD (PER SERVING)		NOTABLE NUTRIENT (PER SERVING)		
Calories	399			
Fat (grams)	7.4		AMOUNT	% DAILY VALUE
% Fat calories	16			
Protein (grams)	35	Calcium (milligrams)	615	61
Carbohydrates (grams)	54			
Cholesterol (milligrams)	33			

1	(12-ounce) package jumbo pasta shells (about 40 shells)
4	cups (32 ounces) fat-free ricotta cheese
½	cup nonfat dried powdered milk
2	tablespoons all-purpose flour
⅛	teaspoon pepper
⅛	teaspoon nutmeg
3	egg whites
8	ounces (2 cups) shredded part-skim mozzarella cheese, divided
½	cup freshly grated Parmesan cheese
1	(26-ounce) jar spaghetti sauce

Prepare the pasta according to the manufacturer's directions. Rinse with cold water and drain.

Meanwhile, using a mixer on low speed, mix together the ricotta cheese, powdered milk, flour, pepper, and nutmeg until blended. Beat in the egg whites. Stir in 1½ cups of the mozzarella and Parmesan cheeses.

Preheat the oven to 350°F. Cover the bottom of a roasting pan with about one third of the spaghetti sauce. Fill the cooked shells with the cheese mixture and arrange in a single layer in the pan. Pour the remaining sauce over the shells. Sprinkle the remaining ½ cup mozzarella cheese. Bake for 30 minutes until bubbly.

Makes 8 servings (about 5 shells each)

Calcium and High Blood Pressure Link

A metaanalysis study reviewing thirty-three studies involving over 2400 people during a thirty-year span found that calcium supplements have little effect on blood pressure in most people. But calcium supplements may help to correct high blood pressure in those with a calcium deficiency.
Journal of the American Medical Association 275(April):1016–1022, 1996

Turkey Divan with Rice

I love this dish because it's an entire meal (dare I say casserole)? To add even more flavor, use rice that has been cooked in chicken broth.

THE SNEAK:

- Nonfat plain yogurt is incorporated into the sauce.
- Nonfat milk is added for the consistency and more calcium.
- A crowning layer of low-fat sharp Cheddar is added for both eye appeal and its bone-building calcium.

NUTRITION SCORECARD (PER SERVING)	
Calories	396
Fat (grams)	9.8
% Fat calories	22
Protein (grams)	37
Carbohydrates (grams)	43
Cholesterol (milligrams)	68

NOTABLE NUTRIENT (PER SERVING)	AMOUNT	% DAILY VALUE
Fiber (grams)	6	24
Calcium (milligrams)	414	41
Vitamin C (milligrams)	85	142

- 1 pound broccoli florets, washed
- 8 ounces turkey tidbits (turkey breast)
- 2 teaspoons curry powder
- 1 (10¾-ounce) can condensed reduced-fat cream of chicken soup
- 1 cup plain nonfat yogurt (without gelatin)
- ¼ cup nonfat milk
- 2 cups cooked brown rice or wild rice
- 1 cup (4 ounces) grated reduced-fat sharp Cheddar cheese

Steam the broccoli just until it turns a vibrant green, about 5 minutes.

Meanwhile, spray a large skillet with nonstick cooking spray. Cook and stir the turkey with the curry powder over medium heat until no longer pink. Set aside.

Preheat the oven to 350°F and spray a 8- × 8-inch or 9- × 9-inch baking pan with nonstick vegetable spray.

In a large bowl stir together the reduced-fat cream soup, yogurt, and milk. Stir in the cooked turkey.

Assemble in layers: Place the cooked rice on the bottom of the pan. Add the cooked broccoli on top of the rice. Pour the turkey mixture evenly over the broccoli. Sprinkle with cheese. Bake for 20 to 25 minutes until golden and bubbly.

Makes 4 entree servings

Calcium Reduces Colon Cancer Risk

Canadian researchers found a 30 percent risk reduction in colon cancer with people whose diets are high in calcium. The protective effect could be due to the formation of calcium soaps, which neutralize the effect of bowel irritation by bile acids and fatty acids. Intervention studies with calcium supplements to reduce colon carcinoma risk are currently under way in Europe.
Cancer 80:858–864, 1997

A naturally occurring fat in cheese called conjugated linoleic acid (CLA) has powerful anti-tumor properties. Blue, Brie, Edam, and Swiss cheeses contain significantly higher CLA.
Cancer 74(August 1):1050–1054, 1994

✖ Swiss and Caraway Fondue ✖

*It doesn't take much of this dip to provide a hefty dose of calcium.
If you don't want to bother with the fondue pot, just use this as
a delicious sauce and serve immediately.*

THE SNEAK:

- Evaporated skim milk is used as the base.
- Low-fat cheese blends nicely into the sauce and provides a rich calcium source without all the fat of regular cheese.

NUTRITION SCORECARD (PER SERVING)		NOTABLE NUTRIENT (PER SERVING)		
Calories	108			
Fat (grams)	3.0		AMOUNT	% DAILY VALUE
% Fat calories	26			
Protein (grams)	10	Calcium (milligrams)	323	32
Carbohydrates (grams)	6			
Cholesterol (milligrams)	13			

¾	cup evaporated skim milk	2	tablespoons dry sherry
1½	teaspoons cornstarch	1½	teaspoons caraway seeds
¾	cup grated reduced-fat Swiss cheese		

Combine 2 teaspoons of the evaporated milk with the cornstarch until smooth. In a small saucepan stir together the cornstarch mixture and the remaining evaporated milk. Cook and stir over medium heat until boiling. Cook for 1 additional minute. Remove from the heat. Stir in the cheese, sherry, and caraway seeds until the cheese melts. Transfer the cheese mixture to a fondue pot; keep the mixture bubbling gently over a fondue burner. Serve with bread cubes or raw vegetables.

Makes 4 servings (about ¼ cup each)

❊ Spicy Cheese Sauce ❊

This sauce makes a nice hot dip for nachos. Pour it over a baked potato or your favorite vegetable.

THE SNEAK:

- Evaporated skim milk is used as the base.
- Nonfat dried powdered milk is added for even more calcium.

NUTRITION SCORECARD (PER SERVING)		NOTABLE NUTRIENT (PER SERVING)		
			AMOUNT	% DAILY VALUE
Calories	131			
Fat (grams)	3.9			
% Fat calories	26			
Protein (grams)	12	Calcium (milligrams)	343	34
Carbohydrates (grams)	13			
Cholesterol (milligrams)	18			

¾	cup evaporated skim milk		¾	cup grated reduced-fat sharp Cheddar cheese
1½	teaspoons cornstarch		½	teaspoon cumin powder
¼	cup nonfat dried powdered milk			
1	(4-ounce) can diced green chilies			

Combine 2 teaspoons of the evaporated milk with the cornstarch until smooth. In a small saucepan stir together the cornstarch mixture, remaining evaporated milk, powdered milk, and green chilies. Cook and stir over medium heat until boiling. Cook for 1 additional minute. Remove from the heat. Stir in the cheese and cumin until the cheese melts. Serve immediately.

Makes 4 servings (about ¼ cup each)

Home-Style Cheddar
✖ Scalloped Potatoes ✖

This is such a winner. Serve this with your favorite green salad and some whole grain bread and you've got yourself a very simple and delicious meal.

THE SNEAK:

- Evaporated skim milk and low-fat cheese kick up the calcium level to almost half of what you need for the entire day!

NUTRITION SCORECARD (PER SERVING)		NOTABLE NUTRIENT (PER SERVING)		
			AMOUNT	% DAILY VALUE
Calories	226			
Fat (grams)	5.3			
% Fat calories	21			
Protein (grams)	17	Calcium (milligrams)	459	46
Carbohydrates (grams)	29			
Cholesterol (milligrams)	24			

4	teaspoons cornstarch	⅛	teaspoon black pepper
1	(12-ounce) can evaporated skim milk	1	cup reduced-fat sharp shredded cheese
⅓	cup chopped onion	3	medium potatoes, peeled and thinly sliced (3 cups)
¼	teaspoon salt		

Preheat the oven to 350°F. Spray a 1-quart casserole with nonstick vegetable spray.

Combine the cornstarch with 2 tablespoons of the milk and stir until smooth. Add the cornstarch mixture, remaining milk, onion, salt, and pepper to a medium saucepan. Cook and stir over medium heat until thickened and bubbly. Cook for 1 additional minute. Remove from the heat and stir in ¾ cup cheese until melted.

Place half of the sliced potatoes into a prepared casserole. Cover with half of the sauce. Repeat layers. Sprinkle the remaining cheese on the top layer.

Bake covered (with a lid or foil) for 35 minutes. Uncover, bake for 30 minutes more until potatoes are tender. Let stand for 5 minutes. Serve.

Makes 4 servings

High Sodium Diets Kick Out Calcium

When sodium is consumed in high amounts, it triggers calcium to be excreted through the urine. This calcium gets robbed from bones, which is why a high sodium diet may decrease bone density and be a contributing factor to osteoporosis. A two-year study of 124 postmenopausal Australian women found that the more sodium a woman consumed (above a teaspoon worth of salt), the greater the loss of bone. Another study in England found a similar relationship in postmenopausal women. The postmenopausal women on high sodium diets had higher bone losses of calcium compared to women on low sodium diets.

European Journal of Clinical Nutrition 51(June):394–399, 1997

❊ Crustless Ricotta-Raspberry Tart ❊

*A layer of ricotta and cream cheese is topped with fresh raspberries
nestled in a thick peach glaze. This refreshing dessert can also double
as a healthy snack—it's one of my family's favorites.*

THE SNEAK:

- A combination of ricotta cheese and fat-free cream cheese gives this
  treat a calcium boost. Fat-free cream cheese has significantly more calcium than regular or light cream cheese.

NUTRITION SCORECARD (PER SERVING)		NOTABLE NUTRIENT (PER SERVING)		
			AMOUNT	% DAILY VALUE
Calories	212			
Fat (grams)	0.2			
% Fat calories	1			
Protein (grams)	16	Calcium (milligrams)	309	31
Carbohydrates (grams)	39			
Cholesterol (milligrams)	14			

1	(8-ounce) package fat-free cream cheese, softened	
1/3	cup sugar	
1	(15-ounce) container fat-free ricotta cheese	
1	(6-ounce) container raspberries, washed	

PEACH GLAZE

1/3 cup sugar
2 tablespoons cornstarch
1 cup peach nectar

In a large bowl, using an electric mixer on low speed, beat together the softened cream cheese and sugar. Fold in the ricotta. Pour the ricotta mixture
into six 8-ounce ramekins. Cover and chill. Meanwhile prepare the glaze.

To make the peach glaze: In a small saucepan combine the sugar and
cornstarch; mix until free from lumps. Add the peach nectar. Cook and
stir over medium heat until thick and bubbly. Remove from the heat. Let
cool for 10 minutes.

To assemble: Place a thin layer of the glaze on top of each ricotta filling (about 1 teaspoon). Arrange the raspberries on top of the thin glaze. Add the remaining glaze over the raspberries. Chill until cool, about 1 hour.

Makes 6 servings

> A high calcium intake helps the body's estrogen work more effectively in protecting the skeleton.
> *American Journal of Clinical Nutrition* 67(1):18–24, 1998

Berry Berry Frozen Yogurt Pie

This is a fast snack or dessert to prepare and it's such a refreshing treat—a favorite for kids. The berries add rich color and flavor.

THE SNEAK:

- A combination of ricotta, nonfat dried milk, and yogurt boosts the calcium to nearly one third of your needs per day.

NUTRITION SCORECARD (PER SERVING)	
Calories	302
Fat (grams)	4.3
% Fat calories	13
Protein (grams)	10
Carbohydrates (grams)	53
Cholesterol (milligrams)	4

NOTABLE NUTRIENT (PER SERVING)	AMOUNT	% DAILY VALUE
Calcium (milligrams)	294	29

2 (8-ounce) containers nonfat berry yogurt (any berry flavor)
1 cup frozen mixed berries (do not thaw)
2/3 cup nonfat dried powdered milk
1/3 cup fat-free ricotta cheese
1/4 cup light corn syrup
2 cups fat-free frozen nondairy whipped topping (thawed)
1 ready-made low-fat graham cracker crust

In a blender combine the yogurt, berries, powdered milk, ricotta, and corn syrup. Blend until smooth with flecks of berries. Gently fold in the thawed whipped topping. Pour the mixture into a graham cracker crust. Cover and freeze until firm, about 4 hours. Remove and let stand at room temperature for 5 to 10 minutes before slicing and serving.

Makes 6 servings (1 pie)

Teen Calcium Shortage

Over 90 percent of teenage girls falls short of the Recommended Dietary Allowance for calcium. Even worse, teens aged fifteen to eighteen consumed less than two thirds of the RDA of this bone-building mineral.
Journal of Adolescent Health 20(Jan.):20–26, 1997

❉ Deep Chocolate Pudding ❉

You'll be scraping the bottom of this dish to get every tasty bit of pudding.

THE SNEAK:

- Using evaporated skim milk, which has twice the calcium content of regular milk
- Incorporating nonfat powdered milk

NUTRITION SCORECARD (PER SERVING)		NOTABLE NUTRIENT (PER SERVING)		
Calories	264			
Fat (grams)	3.7		AMOUNT	% DAILY VALUE
% Fat calories	12			
Protein (grams)	12	Calcium (milligrams)	413	41
Carbohydrates (grams)	49			
Cholesterol (milligrams)	6			

⅔	cup sugar	2	(12-ounce) cans evaporated
⅓	cup cocoa powder		skim milk
¼	cup nonfat dried milk	¼	cup chocolate chips
	powder	1	teaspoon almond extract or
⅓	cup cornstarch		vanilla extract

In a medium saucepan mix together the sugar, cocoa, dried milk, and cornstarch until thoroughly blended with no lumps. Gradually stir in the evaporated milk. Cook and stir over medium heat until boiling and thickened. Cook and stir one additional minute. Remove from the heat and stir in the chocolate chips until melted. Stir in the almond or vanilla extract. Pour into six custard cups. Cover and chill for at least 2 hours until cool.

Makes 6 servings

One McDonald's milk shake provides 35 percent of your calcium needs for the day.
McDonald's Nutrition Facts, February 1997

✳ Home Express Coffee Lattè ✳

This beverage is one of the most popular ways that my clients drink their calcium; it's simplicity at its best. The secret is brewing strong coffee. For a nice variation, try using a flavored brewed coffee such as Irish Cream or hazelnut.

THE SNEAK:

- Heating nonfat milk and adding it to strong coffee

NUTRITION SCORECARD (PER SERVING)		NOTABLE NUTRIENT (PER SERVING)		
			AMOUNT	% DAILY VALUE
Calories	65			
Fat (grams)	0.3			
% Fat calories	5			
Protein (grams)	7	Calcium (milligrams)	228	23
Carbohydrates (grams)	9			
Cholesterol (milligrams)	3			

¾ cup nonfat milk
⅓ cup strong coffee (1½ to double strength)*

dash of cinnamon (optional)

Pour the milk into a large microwavable coffee mug. Microwave on High for about 60 seconds (until hot, but not boiling). Stir in the brewed coffee. Add cinnamon if you wish.

Makes 1 beverage (about 1 cup)

*To make a pot of strong coffee, follow the manufacturer's directions, except increase the amount of coffee grounds by 1½ to twice the amount.

Try these flavorful twists:

- Peppermint Lattè: Add a drop or two of peppermint extract (it's sold where you find vanilla extract).
- Mocha Lattè: Add 2 to 4 teaspoons chocolate syrup (an extra 14 calories per teaspoon).

Is Caffeine a Bone Robber?

Some studies have shown that coffee leaches calcium. To set the record straight once and for all, Penn State researchers recruited 138 healthy post-menopausal women according to their caffeine habits. The researchers found no bone changes (indicated by bone density measurements) whether the women drank zero to eight or more cups of java a day.
  American Journal of Clinical Nutrition 65(June):1826–1830, 1997

Try These Other Calcium-Rich Recipes

Cheddar Chowder	19
Easy Brunch Casserole	217
Enchilada Bake	130
Feta Cheese Dip	95
Florentine Pasta Bundles	105
French Toast Turkey-Ham Sandwiches	177
Home-Style Lasagna	23
Jeff's Thick-Crust Bread-Machine Pizza	151
My Favorite Pinto Beans	127
Three-Pepper Confetti Pasta for Two	21
Turkey Divan with Rice	74
Twice-Baked Potatoes	28

CHAPTER FOUR

The Joy of Soy

Why No Diet Should Be Without

"You're not going to make me a tofu-head are you?" uttered one of my patients as I began to espouse the many benefits of eating soy. My goal in this chapter is not to make you a tofu-head, but to expose you to the many exciting healthy properties of soy and its cousins, followed by some stealthy ways to painlessly incorporate soy into your diet. And if you think that you cannot stand the stuff, I beg you to keep an open mind, for I have fooled many a taste bud (including those of my dear daughter who at one time protested her detestation for tofu and all its kin). Before I get into the culinary aspects of soy (dare I say the joy of soy?), let's first look at what it can do for you and your body.

It's not too often that one food (soy and its products) is held in great esteem by researchers and nutritionists for its role in preventing so many health conditions—from heart disease to the side effects of menopause. While the research on soy's health-promoting properties is still in its infancy, the healing power of soy cannot be denied.

Heart Disease. A landmark study published in the *New England Journal of Medicine* in 1995 catapulted interest in soy into the mainstream. Researchers at the University of Kentucky culled the data from 38 clinical soy protein studies to make one significant size study of 740 participants. Until that time most studies on soy were too small to draw any substantial conclusions. It was found that:

- 84 percent of the studies showed a decrease in the LDL cholesterol (the bad cholesterol) by 13 percent.
- The higher the person's blood cholesterol, the more impact the soy protein had. People who had cholesterol levels higher than 333 milligrams had a 20 percent reduction from eating soy protein.
- Levels of HDL, the protective form or "good" cholesterol, did not change, which is beneficial. (Often when total cholesterol is lowered, the HDL also gets pulled down.)
- The greater the soy protein intake, the greater the drop in cholesterol. Eating 25 grams (almost one ounce) of soy protein resulted in a decrease of 9 milligrams of cholesterol. And eating three times that amount of soy protein (75 grams) resulted in a threefold decrease of 26 milligrams cholesterol.

Keep in mind that (based on the results of this study) only people with high blood cholesterol will see significant results by adding soy protein. People with healthy or borderline-high cholesterol levels probably won't see a drop from added soy, but they may reap other benefits.

Soy protein may reduce the risk of other chronic diseases, including many forms of cancer and osteoporosis. Not to mention that soy may relieve the uncomfortable side effects of menopause. Here's why. Soy is rich in a class of phytoestrogens also known as isoflavones, which can act like hormones in the body.

Menopause. Phytoestrogen compounds in soy (particularly, genistein and daidzein) can mimic estrogen, especially in estrogen-depleted women. In this case, the phytoestrogen acts as a pinch hitter for estrogen, filling in where the body's own hormone would be. Researchers think that phytoestrogen occupies the sites that estrogen would normally occupy (if available) during menopause, resulting in fewer symptoms such as hot flashes. It could be the reason why high-tofu eating cultures, especially Japanese women, have markedly lower discomfort from menopause than women in Western countries.

Cancer. These same biologically active compounds may also play a role in preventing hormone-dependent cancers such as breast cancer, endometrial cancer, and even prostate cancer. Typically cultures that have a high intake of soy, in addition to a low-fat diet (such as the Japanese and Chinese), have a lower risk for breast, uterine, prostate, and colon cancers. Researchers believe that the high level of the estrogenlike isoflavones in soy foods may be the explanation.

Healthy Blood Vessels. Specific phytoestrogens, notably genistein, may guard against heart disease and even migraine headaches through its action in the blood vessels. Genistein interferes with an enzyme (tyrosine kinase) that leads to blood platelet traffic jams (platelet clumping and blood clotting). Therefore, soy may help keep the blood cell pathway smooth and uncluttered.

Bone Health. A very encouraging study by researchers at the University of Illinois looked at the effects of soy (notably isoflavones) on postmenopausal women. At the end of the twenty-four-week experiment, there was a significant increase in bone mineral content and bone density. Of course, more research is needed to confirm these findings, but these results are similar to animal studies that show that soy is a bone protector.

Just remember to keep in mind the nature of research. It must take place step by step. Scientists are still gathering clues on the exact mechanism(s) and the role that soy will play in our future. It's still too early to say exactly how much soy in our diet will offer health protection. But it's comforting to know that, unlike other food compounds and nutrients making nutrition headlines, adding soy to your diet is inherently safe. Many cultures have consumed it for centuries.

GETTING STARTED

There are many ways to add soy into your diet. It can be as simple as taking a stroll down your grocery aisles. No longer is soy relegated to health food stores. More than two thousand new soy products have been introduced since 1985, and even the big food companies such as Green Giant have entered the fray. Refer to Twenty Ways to Increase Soy in Your Diet, page 94, to get ideas on how you can add soy into your diet.

The recipes in this chapter are designed to incorporate soy into familiar meals and dishes—it's not an all or nothing approach. You don't have to give up beef or chicken to gain the benefits of soy, just modify a few of your favorite dishes to include soy products. For example, in the Toasted Tacos Olé recipe, page 101, I used half ground lean beef and half crumbled tofu.

If you or a loved one are afraid to try soy, or perhaps have had a bad experience with it, I suggest beginning with a recipe where soy is totally stealthy, such as in the Chocolate Marble Cheesecake, page 111. In fact, it was a tofu cheesecake that turned my daughter's thinking around, from "gross" to willing to try it in other recipes. Although I must confess that I made the cheesecake without telling her what was in it, I eventually revealed the "secret ingredient" after she had several helpings and pleaded for more!

Five Ways to Sneak Soy into Meals

1. Puree tofu and add it to a cheesecake or custard. For example, see Pumpkin Custard with Gingersnap Crumble, page 109.

2. Crumble tofu and incorporate it into ground meat or ricotta recipes. For example, see Florentine Pasta Bundles, page 105, where the crumbled tofu blends stealthily with the ricotta.

3. Dice tofu and incorporate into recipes containing food with similar shapes, such as Eggcellent Egg Salad Sandwiches, page 99.

4. Infuse tofu. Tofu has a very neutral, bland flavor that takes on the surrounding flavors. For example, see Curly Noodle Soup, page 98, or Tortilla Soup, page 96.

5. Substitute soy products for conventional ones in traditional recipes such as using soy milk in Golden Rice Pudding, page 108.

Soy at a Glance Glossary

Soy products come in many forms. Here's a quick glossary to remove the mystery.

Term	What It Is
Green soybeans	Are harvested just prior to their maturity. They are nestled in a pod, similar in size and color to green peas.
Miso	Fermented soybean paste used often as a flavoring agent or condiment. Can be found in Asian markets, the international aisle of the grocery store, and health food stores.
Soybeans	A legume that comes in many forms: fresh, dry, and sprouted. The seeds yield soy flour, soy milk, and oil (soybean oil).
Soy flour	It has no gluten, therefore it can only be partially substituted for regular flour in recipes—for up to 15 to 20 percent of the total flour amount. Soy flour has double the protein of whole wheat flour.
Soy milk	The extracted liquid made from ground whole soy beans and water. If you are using soy milk in lieu of dairy milk, choose a soy milk that is fortified with calcium. Can be found in most grocery stores.
Soy nuts	Soybeans that have been soaked and roasted.
Tempeh	A fermented soybean product that originated in Indonesia two thousand years ago. Has a rich mushroomlike flavor.
Textured Soy Protein (TSP)	A dehydrated product made from soy flour, also known as textured vegetable protein (TVP). When water is added, TSP takes on the texture of ground meat. It works best in dishes flavored with tomato sauce such as spaghetti.
Tofu	Soybean curd made from soybean milk. The curds are usually made with a coagulating agent (similar to the cheese-making process). When calcium sulfate is used as the coagulant, the tofu has a higher calcium content. Tofu comes in different textures based on its water content. The *firm* and *extra-firm* tofu has less water

Term	What It Is
Tofu (*cont.*)	and is higher in protein. It's best used in recipes in which you want the tofu to retain its shape, such as in stir-fries or for grilling. *Soft* or *silken* tofu has a custardlike texture and gets less coagulant. It blends particularly well and is suited for dips, dressings, and shakes.
Tofu, pressed	Tofu is wrapped in paper towels and placed between two flat surfaces such as cutting boards or cookie sheets. Then it is weighted down by a heavy object such as a brick or your favorite cookbook tome. Water is pressed out, which leads to a firmer tofu. This technique can convert soft tofu into firm tofu.

Soy Foods and Protein

Substituting soy protein for animal protein helps to lower cholesterol. Substantial amounts of phytoestrogens can be obtained by eating 1 to 2 ounces of soy protein daily, which can be found in one half cup tofu, one third cup soy flour, or one cup soy milk.

Soy Source	Serving Size	Soy Protein grams
Basic Soy Products		
Isolated soy protein powder	1 ounce	23
Miso	½ cup	16
Soybeans, mature, boiled	½ cup	14
Soy flour, defatted	½ cup	24
Soy milk	1 cup	4–10
Sprouted soybeans	½ cup	4
Tempeh	½ cup	16
Textured soy protein	½ cup	11
Tofu, firm	½ cup	20
Commercial Products		
Boca Burger, Vegan original	1 (2.5 ounces)	12
Fantastic Foods Shells 'n Curry w/tofu	1 cup	22
Green Giant Breakfast Links	3 links (2.4 ounces)	12
Green Giant Harvest Burger, original	1 (3.2 ounces)	18
Legume Classic Enchiladas	2 (11 ounces)	16
Legume Vegetable Lasagna	11 ounces	16
Lightlife Smart Dogs	1 (1.5 ounces)	9

Twenty Ways to Increase Soy in Your Diet

1. Add crumbled tofu to scrambled eggs.
2. Mix half pureed tofu with half low-fat ricotta and use in your favorite lasagna or manicotti recipe.
3. Try using calcium-fortified soy milk with your favorite pudding mix.
4. Add diced tofu to your favorite potato salad recipe.
5. Puree tofu and blend it with your favorite dip mix such as onion or ranch style.
6. Substitute pureed tofu for mayonnaise in your favorite dressing mix.
7. Top your salad with roasted soy nuts.
8. Add diced tofu to your favorite broth-based soup such as minestrone.
9. Add crumbled tofu to your favorite casserole such as tuna noodle or macaroni and cheese.
10. Try at least one new soy convenience product a week, from sausage links to soy cheese.
11. Marinate tofu chunks in teriyaki sauce or your favorite dressing and keep on hand for an easy snack.
12. Throw extra-firm tofu or tempeh on the grill.
13. Cut a thin slice of baked tofu (a convenience product) and add it to your favorite sandwich.
14. Skewer extra-firm tofu chunks when making shish kabobs.
15. Add soy nuts to your favorite cookie or brownie recipe.
16. Try a traditionally prepared soy food in a restaurant such as Japanese miso soup. (Miso is fermented soybean paste.)
17. Try a new twist on your favorite meat loaf. Combine 1/2 meatless sausage (soy-based) with half lean ground meat.
18. Replace one third to one half of the cream cheese with pureed tofu in a cheesecake recipe.
19. Try one new soy recipe a week. (This chapter is a good beginning!)
20. Use pureed tofu in Twice-Baked Potatoes, page 28. Scoop out the baked potato pulp and combine with the tofu. Refill the potato shell with tofu mixture, top with low-fat shredded cheese, and bake again until melted.

✖ Feta Cheese Dip ✖

This savory dip is a crowd pleaser; no one will guess that there is tofu in here!

THE SNEAK:

- Tofu is crumbled and mixed together with the strongly flavored Feta cheese.

NUTRITION SCORECARD (PER SERVING)		NOTABLE NUTRIENT (PER SERVING)		
Calories	69			
Fat (grams)	2.3		AMOUNT	% DAILY VALUE
% Fat calories	30			
Protein (grams)	8	Calcium (milligrams)	299	30
Carbohydrates (grams)	3			
Cholesterol (milligrams)	15			

4	ounces low-fat firm tofu	2	teaspoons grated onion	
2	ounces Feta cheese	2	teaspoons dried dillweed	
1	(8-ounce) tub fat-free cream cheese	1	teaspoon white wine vinegar	
1	tablespoon snipped parsley	¼	teaspoon coarse black pepper	
2	cloves garlic, minced	⅛	teaspoon paprika	

Crumble the tofu and place in a medium bowl. Using a fork, stir and crumble the Feta cheese until thoroughly mixed. Add the fat-free cream cheese, parsley, garlic, onion, dillweed, vinegar, black pepper, and paprika. Using an electric mixer beat the mixture on low speed until blended. Cover and chill until ready to serve.

Serving suggestion: Serve with whole grain crackers or crisp pita bread wedges.

Makes 6 servings (1⅔ cups)

✳ Tortilla Soup ✳

It's hard to believe that a soup this tasty is so easy to make. You might want to throw in a few more tortilla strips into the oven—they make a great snack. Baked tofu is a product that you can purchase in the deli section of the grocery store or at health food stores. It has a firmer, heartier texture than regular tofu; it is firmly pressed, then baked.

THE SNEAK:

- Tiny baked tofu cubes are infused with a pleasant Southwest flavor. This particular baked tofu has a head start with its built-in savory flavor.

NUTRITION SCORECARD (PER SERVING)	
Calories	294
Fat (grams)	7.8
% Fat calories	23
Protein (grams)	27
Carbohydrates (grams)	31
Cholesterol (milligrams)	10

4 cups fat-free chicken broth
1 cup chopped onion
2 cloves garlic, minced
1 (4-ounce) can diced green chile
½ teaspoon cumin powder
12 ounces savory flavor baked tofu, diced
¼ cup chopped cilantro

TORTILLA STRIPS
nonstick vegetable spray
4 corn tortillas
2 tomatoes, chopped
4 tablespoons shredded reduced-fat sharp Cheddar

In a large saucepan combine the chicken broth, onion, garlic, chile, and cumin. Bring to a boil. Reduce the heat and add the baked tofu and cilantro. Cover and simmer for 15 minutes. Meanwhile, prepare the tortilla strips.

To make the tortilla strips: Preheat the oven to 375°F. Spray a baking sheet with nonstick vegetable spray. Cut the tortillas in half and then into short ¹/₂-inch strips. Place them in a single layer on the baking sheet. Spray the strips with nonstick spray (this will help them crisp). Bake for 10 minutes until golden brown.

To assemble the soup: Divide the soup among four bowls. Add the tortilla chips, tomatoes, and cheese to each bowl. Serve immediately.

Makes 4 servings (1¹/₂ cups each)

Genistein

Estrogens can stimulate the growth of breast tumors in experimental animal studies. But genistein, a phytoestrogen in soy can function as an antagonist—tricking the body into producing less estrogen. This competitive mechanism may reduce the risk of estrogen-sensitive tumors such as breast cancer. One half cup soybeans, 1 cup soy beverage, or 4 ounces of tofu provide 30 to 40 milligrams of genistein.
Journal of the American Dietetic Association 97(10 supplement 2):s201, 1997

Over thirty laboratory studies show that genistein, one of two key phytoestrogens in soy, has the ability to inhibit the growth of cancer cells.
Environmental Nutrition 17(5):1, 4 1994

Curly Noodle Soup

The long curly fusilli noodles add a delightful twist to this Asian-flavored soup. Don't skimp on the sesame oil here; its flavor is too important and its absence would surely be missed. Besides, the amount of oil added is very small. Adding the greens at the very end of the soup helps to preserve heat-sensitive nutrients.

THE SNEAK:

- The little cubes of tofu absorb the strong aromatic flavors (fresh ginger, toasted sesame oil). The tofu's soft texture melds with the texture of the pasta.

NUTRITION SCORECARD (PER SERVING)	
Calories	204
Fat (grams)	4.6
% Fat calories	20
Protein (grams)	14
Carbohydrates (grams)	27
Cholesterol (milligrams)	0

- 4 cups fat-free chicken broth
- 2 cups sliced shiitake mushrooms or other sliced mushrooms
- 3 tablespoons reduced-salt soy sauce
- 1 tablespoon grated fresh ginger
- 3 cloves garlic, minced
- 1/8 teaspoon red chili flakes
- 1 (12-ounce) package low-fat silken firm tofu, diced
- 4 ounces fusilli noodles (or a curly noodle such as rotelle)
- 4 cups snipped bok choy greens or spinach
- 1/2 cup snipped chives
- 2 teaspoons sesame oil

In a large 4-quart pan combine the broth, mushrooms, soy sauce, ginger, garlic, and red chili flakes. Bring to a boil. Reduce the heat. Add the tofu and cover the pan. Cook until the vegetables are tender, about 5 minutes. Bring the soup to a boil and carefully add the noodles. Cook, covered, stirring occasionally, until the noodles are tender, about 10 minutes. Stir in the bok choy greens and cook until just wilted and vibrant green. Remove from the heat. Stir in the chives and sesame oil. Serve immediately.

Makes 4 servings (1 1/2 cups each)

Chinese who regularly consume soybeans and/or tofu have only 50 percent the incidence of cancer of the stomach, colon, rectum, breast, and lung as those Chinese who rarely consume soy products.
Journal of the American Dietetic Association 97(10 supplement 2):s201, 1997

✖ Eggcellent Egg Salad Sandwiches ✖

I love egg salad sandwiches, especially these in which the cholesterol is lowered significantly by using tofu, but you wouldn't know it by looking at or tasting it.

THE SNEAK:

- Replace some of the whole eggs with tofu—the diced tofu resembles hard-cooked egg whites.
- Dry mustard powder is added for its yellow color and flavor.

NUTRITION SCORECARD (PER SERVING)		NOTABLE NUTRIENT (PER SERVING)		
Calories	213			
Fat (grams)	5.9		AMOUNT	% DAILY VALUE
% Fat calories	24			
Protein (grams)	12.2	Fiber (grams)	4	16
Carbohydrates (grams)	29			
Cholesterol (milligrams)	107			

3	eggs	1	tablespoon fat-free cream
4	ounces light silken tofu,		cheese
	extra firm	¼	teaspoon vinegar
¼	cup finely chopped chives	½	teaspoon dry mustard powder
2	tablespoons finely chopped	¼	teaspoon salt
	green pepper	⅛	teaspoon black pepper
2	tablespoons low-fat	8	slices whole wheat bread
	mayonnaise		

Place the eggs in a small saucepan. Add enough *cold* water to cover the eggs. Bring to a boil over high heat. Reduce heat so the water is just below simmering. Cook for 15 minutes. Drain. To cool eggs quickly, fill the saucepan with cold water and let stand 2 or more minutes. Peel the eggshells. Cut the eggs in half and discard one of the yolks.

While the eggs are cooking, wrap the tofu with a paper towel and gently press out any excess liquid. Dice the tofu into small cubes about the size of a pea and place in a medium bowl. Add the chives and chopped green pepper.

In a small bowl stir together the mayonnaise, fat-free cream cheese, vinegar, dry mustard powder, salt, and pepper. Crumble the egg yolk into the mayonnaise mixture. Stir until smooth.

Chop the egg whites and mix into the tofu mixture. Add the mayonnaise mixture and stir until well blended. Divide the egg mixture on four slices of bread. Top with the remaining bread slices.

Makes 4 whole sandwiches

�֎ Toasted Tacos Olé ✖

*I watched my daughter eat two of these tacos and ask for a third;
she had no idea that the filling contained tofu.*

THE SNEAK:

- Uses half ground meat and half crumbled tofu, topped with the traditional accoutrements—who would know? The small amount of cocoa powder adds a nice brown color.
- Bonus sneak—corn tortillas are crisped in the toaster and used instead of conventional fried taco shells to reduce fat.

```
NUTRITION SCORECARD
(PER SERVING—2 TACOS)

Calories              290
Fat (grams)             8.7
% Fat calories         26
Protein (grams)        18
Carbohydrates
   (grams)             37
Cholesterol
   (milligrams)        31
```

8	ounces low-fat firm tofu	3	tablespoons water
1	cup chopped onion	12	corn tortillas
3	cloves garlic, minced	½	cup finely shredded low-fat Cheddar cheese
½	teaspoon cocoa powder	2	cups shredded lettuce
8	ounces extra-lean ground beef	2	tomatoes, diced
1	(1¼ ounces) package taco seasoning		salsa (optional)

Spray a large skillet with nonstick vegetable spray. Using your fingers, crumble the tofu into tiny pieces (resembling cottage cheese) and add to the skillet along with the onion, garlic, and cocoa powder. Cook and stir over medium heat until the onion is translucent. Add the ground beef and cook until no longer pink, about 10 minutes. Sprinkle the taco seasoning mixture and the water over the crumbled tofu mixture. Stir to mix thoroughly. Reduce heat to low and cover.

Meanwhile, toast the corn tortillas in a toaster until golden. Spoon about 3 tablespoons of the tofu filling into the toasted taco shells. Top with cheese, lettuce, tomatoes, and salsa if desired.

Makes 12 tacos, 6 servings (2 tacos each)

Tofu a Protective Factor for Breast Cancer

A protective effect of tofu was observed in a case control study of Asian-American women. The more tofu eaten, the greater the decrease in risk of breast cancer. Asian-American women who were born in Asia had twice the tofu intake (sixty-two times per year) as compared to Asians born in the U.S. The immigrants' intake of tofu decreased with years of residence in the U.S. This may explain why breast cancer rates of Asian Americans are lower than those of U.S. Caucasians but considerably higher than the rates in Asia.

Wu A. et al. *Tofu and risk of breast cancer in Asian-Americans. Cancer Epidemiology, Biomarkers and Prevention* 5(Nov.):901–906, 1996

✖ Meatless Patties ✖

Veggie burgers are rising in popularity; they are served at many restaurants and are even popping up in traditional grocery stores. Because of this trend I have found people to be very receptive to this recipe. I just tell them it's a meatless burger. It is very simple to make and a family favorite.

THE SNEAK:

• Tofu is crumbled into a mixture that works surprisingly well.

NUTRITION SCORECARD (PER SERVING)	
Calories	214
Fat (grams)	4.9
% Fat calories	20
Protein (grams)	12
Carbohydrates (grams)	32
Cholesterol (milligrams)	0

1 (12-ounce) package low-fat firm tofu
2 egg whites, lightly beaten
1 package instant onion soup mix

1 cup oatmeal
6 whole wheat hamburger buns
6 romaine lettuce leaves
1 tomato

In a medium bowl crumble the tofu. Stir in the egg whites and onion soup. Add the oats and mix well. Let stand for 5 minutes. Using about ⅓ cup measure for each, shape into 6 patties about ½ inch thick. Spray a griddle or skillet with nonstick vegetable spray. Cook the patties for 3 minutes on each side until golden. Transfer to a hamburger bun. Serve with lettuce and tomato. If desired add other "burger condiments" such as catsup and mustard.

Makes 6 servings

Endometrial Cancer

A study by the Cancer Research Center of Hawaii has found that women who ate the highest amounts of phytoestrogen foods (primarily soy foods) had a 54 percent reduction in endometrial cancer risk.

American Journal of Epidemiology 146(Aug. 15):294–306, 1997

Chili Surprise

It looks like chili, it tastes like chili—so what's the catch? The specks of "ground meat" are in actuality browned tofu. If you want to be extra stealthy, garnish liberally with chives and low-fat cheese.

THE SNEAK:

- Tofu is crumbled and browned, which resembles ground meat in the chili.

NUTRITION SCORECARD (PER SERVING)	
Calories	260
Fat (grams)	2.8
% Fat calories	2.8
Protein (grams)	16
Carbohydrates (grams)	45
Cholesterol (milligrams)	0

NOTABLE NUTRIENT (PER SERVING)	AMOUNT	% DAILY VALUE
Fiber (grams)	11	44
Folic acid (micrograms)	142	36
Iron (milligrams)	3.9	22

1 (12-ounce) package low-fat, firm tofu
2 teaspoons chili powder
1 cup chopped onion
3 cloves garlic, minced
1 green bell pepper, diced
3 (14 ½-ounce) cans pinto beans, rinsed and drained
1 (14 ½-ounce) can diced tomatoes
1 cup salsa
1 tablespoon ground cumin
1 tablespoon Worcestershire sauce

Optional Garnishes:

chopped fresh tomatoes
shredded low-fat Cheddar cheese

Preheat the oven to 350°F.

Spray a baking sheet with nonstick vegetable spray. Using your fingers, crumble the tofu into tiny pieces and spread over a baking sheet. Sprinkle the chili powder over the crumbled tofu and stir to mix thoroughly. Bake for 30 minutes, stirring occasionally. Remove from the oven.

Meanwhile, spray a large 4-quart saucepan with nonstick vegetable spray. Add the onion, garlic, and bell pepper. Cook and stir over medium heat until the onion is translucent, about 5 minutes. Add the pinto beans, tomatoes, salsa, cumin, and Worcestershire sauce. Bring to a boil. Reduce the heat to a simmer and cover. Stir in the baked tofu and simmer with the lid on for 45 minutes or longer.

Divide the chili into six bowls. Garnish if desired with tomatoes and low-fat Cheddar cheese.

Makes 6 servings

✖ Florentine Pasta Bundles ✖

Freshly grated Parmesan cheese is the key to this flavorful dish.
For a Mediterranean flair, try using crumbled Feta cheese instead of
Parmesan cheese.

THE SNEAK:

- Tofu is crumbled and discreetly tucked inside a rolled-up lasagna noodle between the spinach and Parmesan cheese.

NUTRITION SCORECARD (PER SERVING—2 BUNDLES)		NOTABLE NUTRIENT (PER SERVING—2 BUNDLES)		
Calories	388			
Fat (grams)	7.9		AMOUNT	% DAILY VALUE
% Fat calories	18			
Protein (grams)	28	Vitamin A (RE)	1333	133
Carbohydrates		Folic Acid (micrograms)	157	39
(grams)	54	Calcium (milligrams)	504	50
Cholesterol				
(milligrams)	16			

8	lasagna noodles	⅔	cup fresh grated Parmesan cheese
1	cup chopped onion		
4	cloves garlic, minced	1½	cups low-fat commercial spaghetti sauce
2	teaspoons dried basil		
12	ounces low-fat tofu, firm, crumbled	½	cup shredded reduced-fat mozzarella cheese (do not use fat-free), divided
2	(10-ounce) packages frozen chopped spinach, thawed and drained		

Cook the noodles according to the manufacturer's directions; rinse and drain. Coat a large skillet with nonstick olive oil spray. Over medium heat, sauté the onion, garlic, basil, and crumbled tofu until the onion is translucent, about 5 minutes. Add the drained spinach and Parmesan cheese. Cook and stir until the cheese begins to melt, about 5 minutes.

Place enough spaghetti sauce to form a thin layer on the bottom of a 12- × 7-inch baking dish. Preheat the oven to 350°F.

On a sheet of wax paper, place one cooked noodle. Add the spinach mixture to ¼-inch border of noodle. Sprinkle about 1½ teaspoons of mozzarella cheese. Roll up like a burrito and place seam side down in a prepared baking dish. Repeat with the remaining noodles. Top lasagna roll-ups with the remaining sauce and sprinkle with the remaining mozzarella cheese. Bake, covered with foil for 35 to 45 minutes, until bubbly.

Makes 8 bundles. Serves 4

Fewer Hot Flashes with Soy

In a study at Bowman Gray School of Medicine in North Carolina, women who were experiencing hot flashes reported less severe symptoms when they added 20 grams of powdered soy protein to their diet.
Environmental Nutrition 20(2):8, 1997

❋ Teriyaki Stir-fry ❋

Fresh ginger with an accent of sesame oil makes this a fragrant dish that you will want to make over and over again.

THE SNEAK:

• Tofu cubes are marinated in a teriyaki sauce that infuses delightful flavor and changes the color to a caramel brown.

NUTRITION SCORECARD (PER SERVING)		NOTABLE NUTRIENT (PER SERVING)		
Calories	177			
Fat (grams)	2.5		AMOUNT	% DAILY VALUE
% Fat calories	13			
Protein (grams)	10	Fiber (grams)	4	16
Carbohydrates		Vitamin A (RE)	1091	109
(grams)	27	Vitamin C (milligrams)	67	112
Cholesterol				
(milligrams)	0			

TERIYAKI MARINADE

⅓ cup lite soy sauce
¼ cup dry sherry
¼ cup packed brown sugar
2 tablespoons pineapple juice
2 teaspoons freshly grated
    ginger
1 clove garlic, minced
1 teaspoon toasted sesame
    seed oil (dark brown color)

⅛ teaspoon chili flakes
12 ounces low-fat tofu, extra firm,
    cut into ½-inch cubes
2 carrots, cut into thin strips
    about 2 inches long
2 cups broccoli florets
1 cup Chinese pea pods
1 teaspoon cornstarch

In a small shallow pan combine the soy sauce, dry sherry, brown sugar, pineapple juice, ginger, garlic, sesame oil, and chili flakes. Add the tofu cubes. Cover and chill. Marinate for at least 1 hour or overnight. Drain the tofu, but *reserve* the marinade.

In a large skillet add about 2 tablespoons of the marinade. Add the tofu. Cook and gently stir over medium-high heat for 3 minutes. Remove the tofu from the pan and set in a bowl or plate. Carefully add 2 more tablespoons of the marinade and carrots. Cook and stir for 2 minutes. Add 2 more tablespoons of the marinade and broccoli. Cook and stir for 2 minutes. Add the Chinese pea pods.

Combine the cornstarch with the remaining marinade and add to the skillet. Cook and stir until bubbly. Reduce the heat. Add the tofu to the pan and cook until heated through, about 1 minute. Serve over rice if desired.

Makes 4 servings

Hot flashes, a typical symptom of menopause in Western women, are such infrequent symptoms in Japan that there is no Japanese word or phrase for it.
Environmental Nutrition 20(2):8, 1997

Golden Rice Pudding

My kids love this treat for an afternoon snack. This pudding has a rich brown color mostly from the vanilla soy milk.

THE SNEAK:

- Vanilla soy milk is used in place of traditional milk.

NUTRITION SCORECARD (PER SERVING)	
Calories	288
Fat (grams)	2.3
% Fat calories	7
Protein (grams)	6
Carbohydrates (grams)	62
Cholesterol (milligrams)	0

1	large package (six-serving size) vanilla pudding mix (not instant)	3	cups cooked brown rice
		⅓	cup golden raisins
3	cups vanilla soy milk	¾	teaspoon cinnamon

In a large saucepan combine the vanilla pudding mix and vanilla soy milk. Cook and stir constantly until the mixture reaches a full boil. Remove from the heat. Stir in the cooked rice, raisins, and cinnamon. Spoon into dessert dishes. Serve warm or chilled.

Makes 6 servings (¾ cup each)

Pumpkin Custard
✖ with Gingersnap Crumble ✖

This makes an outstanding snack and a great introduction to tofu—one of my favorites.

THE SNEAK:

• Tofu is pureed and mixed into pumpkin. The presence of tofu is undetectable!

NUTRITION SCORECARD (PER SERVING)		NOTABLE NUTRIENT (PER SERVING)		
Calories	216			
Fat (grams)	3.6		AMOUNT	% DAILY VALUE
% Fat calories	15			
Protein (grams)	7	Vitamin A (RE)	1576	158
Carbohydrates (grams)	40			
Cholesterol (milligrams)	5			

12	ounces low-fat tofu, firm, drained	½	teaspoon cloves
1	(15-ounce) can pumpkin (1¾ cups)	3	egg whites
⅔	cup packed brown sugar		
1	teaspoon rum extract		
1½	teaspoons cinnamon		
¾	teaspoon ginger		

GINGERSNAP TOPPING

8	gingersnap cookies
1	tablespoon white sugar
2	tablespoons light butter

To make the pumpkin custard: Preheat the oven to 350°F. Spray six 6-ounce custard cups with nonstick vegetable spray. In a food processor or blender puree the tofu until smooth. Add the pumpkin, brown sugar, rum extract, cinnamon, ginger, and cloves. Puree until blended. Add the egg whites and mix just until blended (do not overmix). Divide the pumpkin mixture among the six custard cups. Bake for 20 minutes. Meanwhile prepare the topping. Remove the custard cups from the oven and sprinkle the gingersnap topping over the pumpkin mixture. Return to the oven and bake an additional 20 minutes until the edges of the custard separate from the cups.

To make the gingersnap topping: In a small bowl stir together the gingersnap crumbs and sugar. Using a grater, shred the light butter and add it to the gingersnap mixture. Using a pastry blender or two knives, cut in the light butter until the mixture resembles coarse crumbs.

Makes 6 servings (about ½ cup each)

Soy a Bone Protector?

If animal studies are any indication, soy may play a role in preventing the bone-thinning disease, osteoporosis. Rats with a simulated osteoporosis condition were fed either a high soybean or regular diet. The rats on the high soybean diet had a significantly higher bone density. Researchers believe that bone-protecting properties are either from the soy protein or the isoflavones present in soy.

Journal of Nutrition 126(1):161–167, 1996

✄ Chocolate Marble Cheesecake ✄

One of my favorite ways to introduce someone to tofu is by blending it into a cheesecake. I never reveal the ingredients in this incredible cheesecake until after someone tastes it. In fact, it was tofu-based cheesecake that opened my daughter's eyes to soy products. Up until then, she would only roll her eyeballs at the mere mention of tofu.

Note: Do plan ahead for this cheesecake as it needs to chill thoroughly. I like to make the cheesecake the day before I plan to serve it so that I can refrigerate it overnight.

THE SNEAK:

- Tofu is used in place of some of the cream cheese.

NUTRITION SCORECARD (PER SERVING)		
Calories	207	
Fat (grams)	4.3	
% Fat calories	19	
Protein (grams)	12	
Carbohydrates (grams)	26	
Cholesterol (milligrams)	12	

8	chocolate wafer cookies, crushed	2	tablespoons all-purpose flour
1	cup nonfat cottage cheese	4	egg whites
12	ounces low-fat firm tofu, silken	1	teaspoon vanilla
1	(8-ounce) package light cream cheese (do not use fat-free), at room temperature	¼	cup cocoa powder
		1	teaspoon almond extract
¾	cup plus 2 tablespoons sugar	1	teaspoon instant espresso coffee powder or instant coffee

Preheat the oven to 375°F. Lightly coat a 9-inch springform pan with non-stick vegetable spray. Sprinkle the chocolate cookie crumbs evenly on the bottom of the pan.

In a food processor or blender puree the cottage cheese until smooth and creamy. Add the tofu and pulse until the mixture is creamy. Add the cream cheese, sugar, and flour. Pulse until blended. Add the egg whites and vanilla, pulse just until blended (take care not to overmix the egg whites or the cheesecake is more likely to crack).

Transfer half of the filling to a bowl; stir in the cocoa, remaining 2 tablespoons sugar, almond extract, and espresso powder until well combined.

Pour half of each batter mixture into the crust. Then repeat, pouring the remaining half of each batter into the crust. Using a small knife, gently swirl the two batters.

Bake for 35 to 40 minutes longer until a knife inserted in the center comes out clean. Transfer to a rack and let cool completely, then cover and refrigerate.

To serve, run a knife around the sides of the pan to loosen the cake. Release the pan sides. Cut into wedges.

Makes 8 servings

How Do You Spell "Relief"?

Soy may help relieve migraines according to preliminary results presented at the International Symposium on Soy in Brussels, 1996. Yale University School of Medicine researchers gave migraine sufferers 29 grams of soy protein twice a day for three months. Half of the patients experienced complete relief during the experiment.

Prevention Online, February 1997

CHAPTER FIVE

Full of Beans

Benefits of Nature's Magical Legume

Snicker if you must. Beans really are the magical legume when it comes to nutrition. They are abundantly rich in nutrients that Americans typically lack in their diet: folic acid, an important B vitamin that you'll read more about here; fiber; and iron. They are also loaded in potassium and offer a good source of protein. Yet when you look at the Food Pyramid, beans garner only an honorable mention in the "meat" group. You would be doing your body a healthy favor if you moved beans to the center of your cuisine or at least as a regular side dish. Back in 1990, the California Department of Health recognized the nutritional importance of beans by recommending that every Californian eat beans at least three times a week.

To be clear here, the beans I'm referring to are dried beans, legumes such as lentils, pinto beans, and so forth. These are starchy, hearty beans, loaded in fiber—not the wax bean or green string bean varieties.

Nature's Nutritional Medicine Chest

I will focus on two exceptional nutritional assets of dried beans—fiber and folic acid.

FIBER

Fiber is so important that I've addressed it in a chapter unto itself. But I could not write about the health merits of beans without noting what a substantial payload of fiber they offer. Average Americans meet barely half of their fiber needs each day (averaging 12 grams of fiber for women and 18 for men). Adding only one cup of beans per day would nearly double the national intake average of fiber and place the average person within the recommended level of 25 to 35 grams of fiber per day.

One bowl of beans has more fiber than your basic high fiber cereal—and it's mainly soluble fiber, the type of fiber that's effective in reducing cholesterol.

Studies have demonstrated that beans (even canned pork and beans) lower cholesterol in three to four weeks when given to people with high cholesterol levels. Most researchers attribute the cholesterol-lowering effect of beans to its high fiber content. In fact, one early study showed that beans were just as effective in lowering serum cholesterol as oat bran.

Take a look at Beans: A Nutritional Powerhouse, page 118, and you'll get an appreciation not only for the fiber that beans have to offer but their other nutrients.

FOLIC ACID

While folic acid (also known as folate) was discovered in the 1940s, only in the last five years or so have researchers discovered how important this essential vitamin is to health. Folic acid is undoubtedly important in preventing birth defects, may play a significant role in preventing heart disease, and may play a role in offsetting depression. Let's take a closer look.

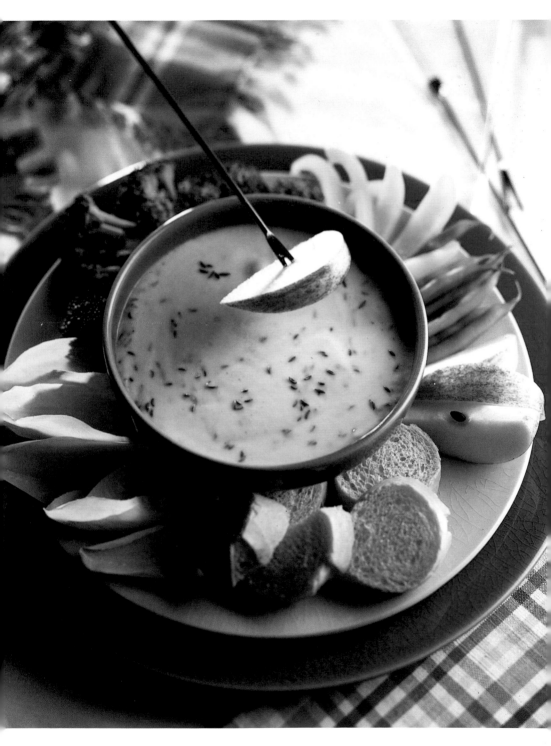

Swiss and Caraway Fondue (page 76)

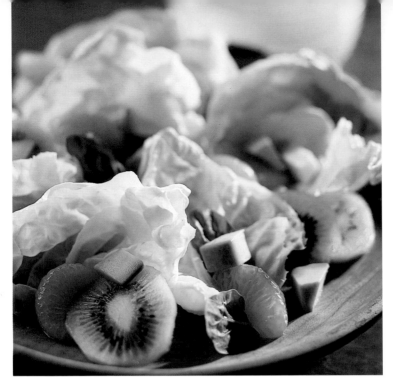

Easy Kiwi
Salad with
Walnut
Vinaigrette
(page 47)

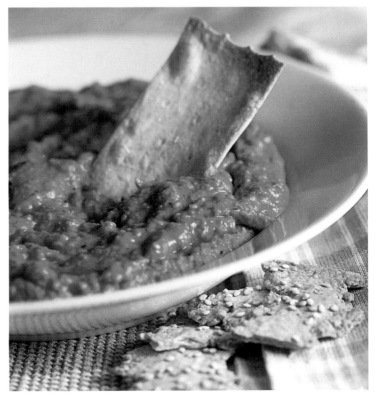

Red Pepper
Hummus with
Roasted Garlic
(page 121)

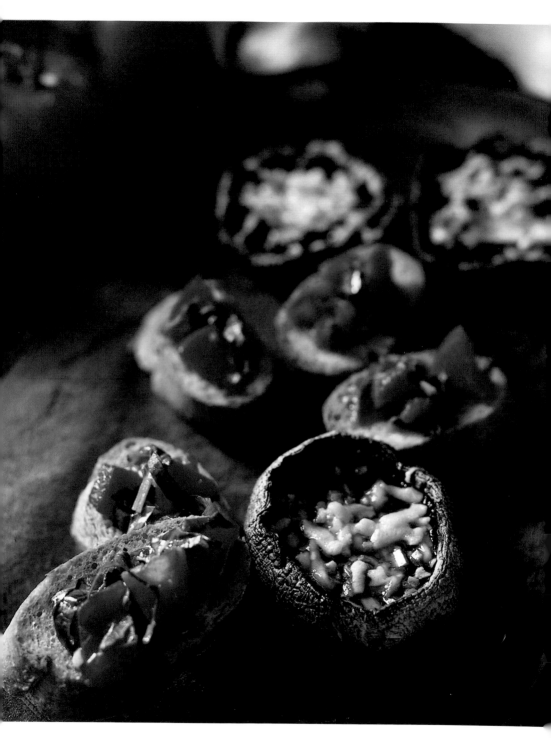

Italian Salsa (page 34) and Garlicky Portobello Mushrooms (page 29)

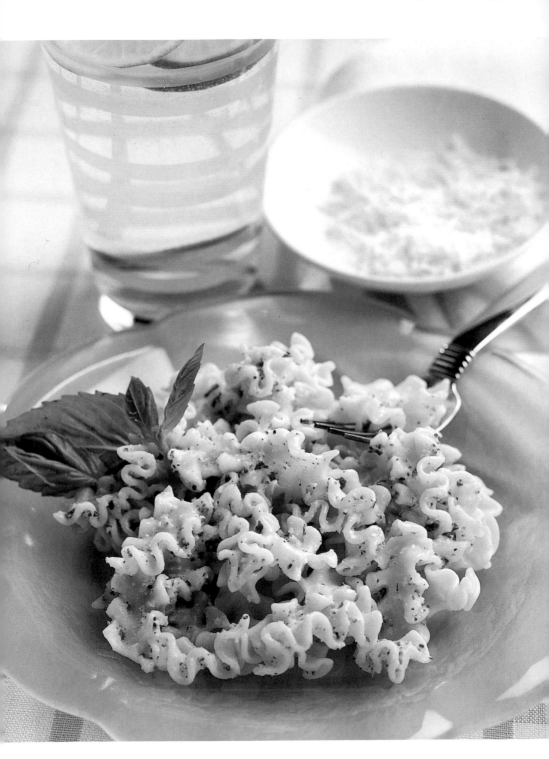

✳ Pesto Pasta Surprise (page 25)

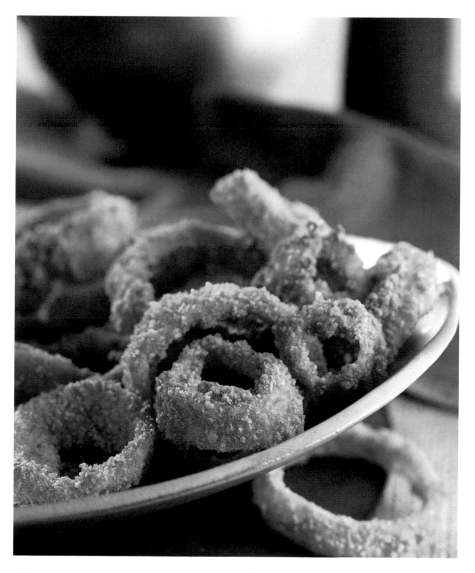

Onion Rings (Practically Fat Free) (page 214)

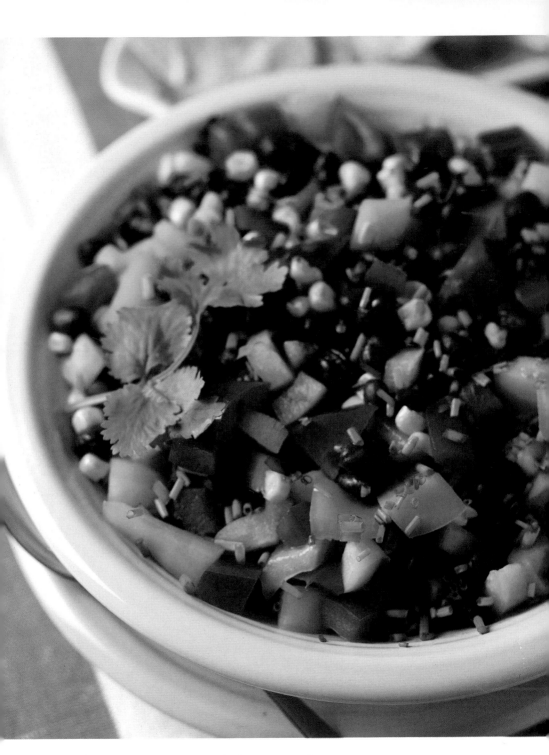

❋ Fiesta Black Bean Salad (page 132)

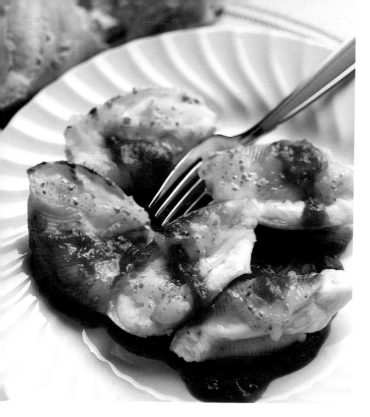

Cheesy Stuffed
Shells
(page 72)

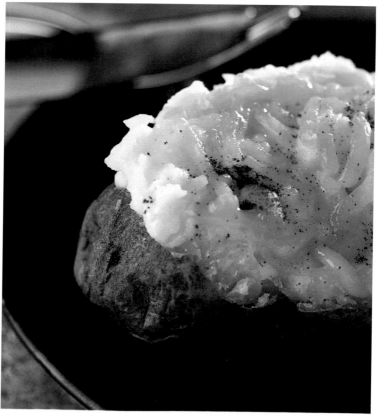

Twice-Baked
Potatoes
(page 28)

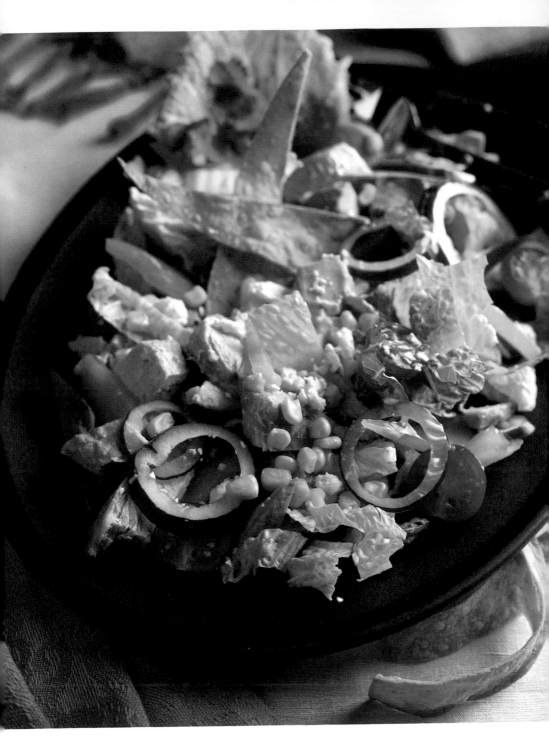

Chicken Salad with Creamy Lime–Cilantro Vinaigrette (page 203)

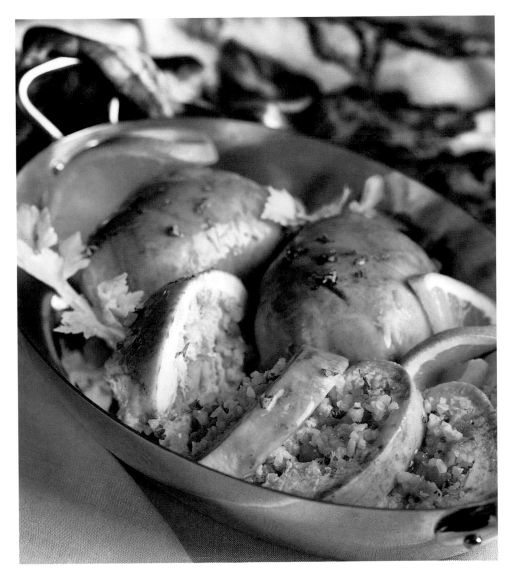

✻ Chicken Bundles with Apricot Stuffing and Honey-Orange Sauce
(page 161)

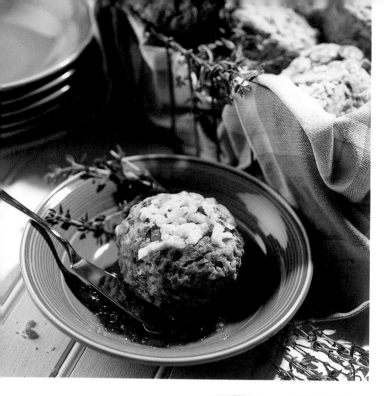

Herbed Biscuits
(page 154)

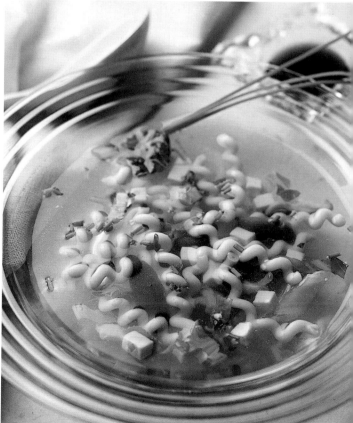

Curly Noodle Soup
(page 98)

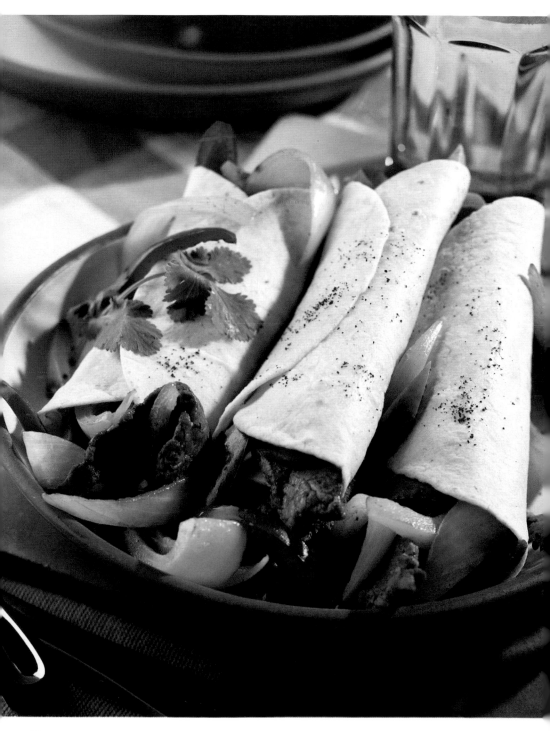

Fiesta Fajitas (page 179)

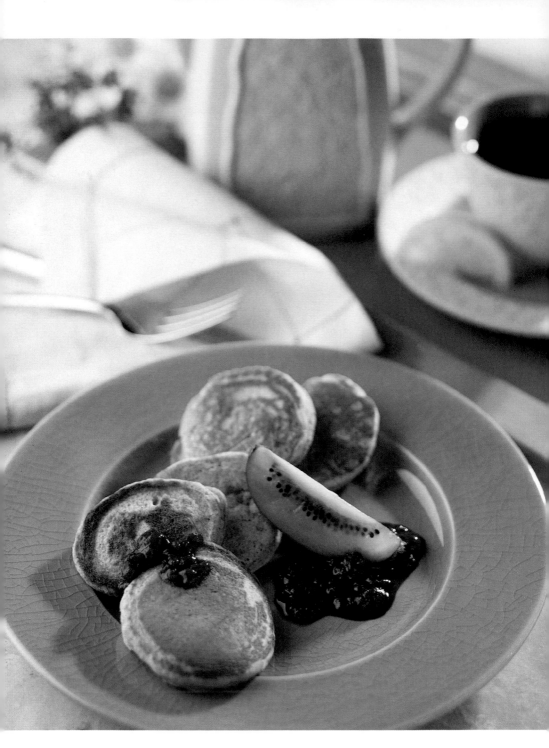

Silver Dollar Pancakes with Rowdy Raspberry Sauce (page 145)

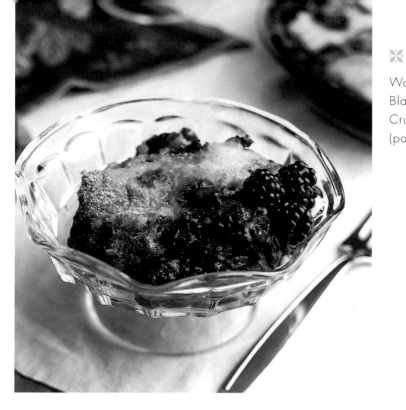

Warm
Blackberry
Crustless Pie
(page 53)

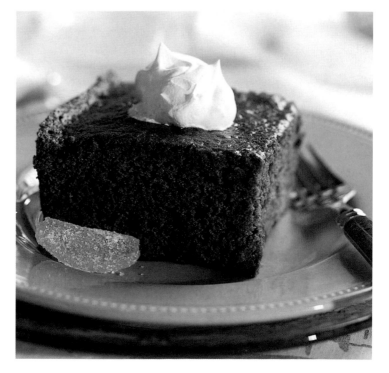

Spiced
Gingerbread
(page 190)

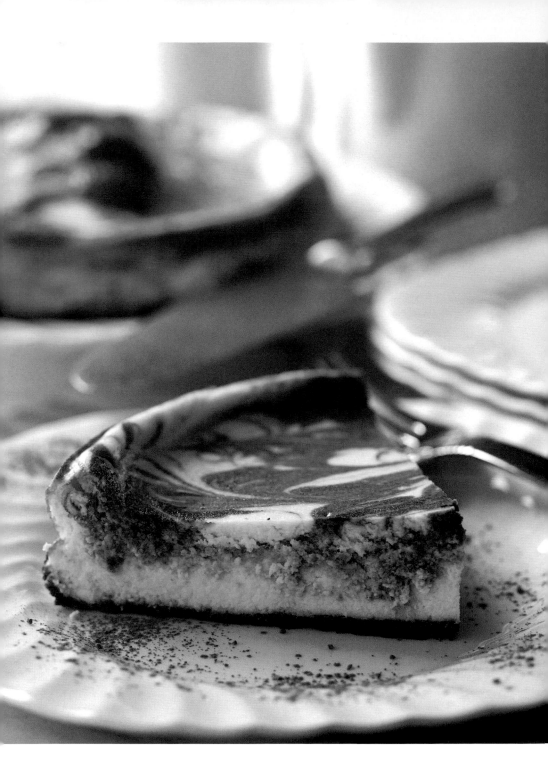

✳ Chocolate Marble Cheesecake (page 111)

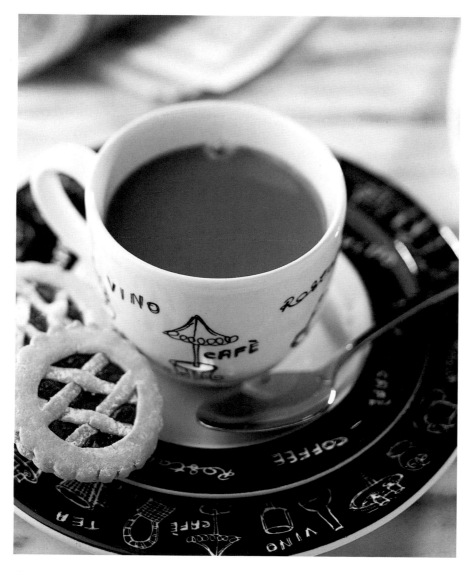

�֎ Home Express Coffee Lattè (page 84)

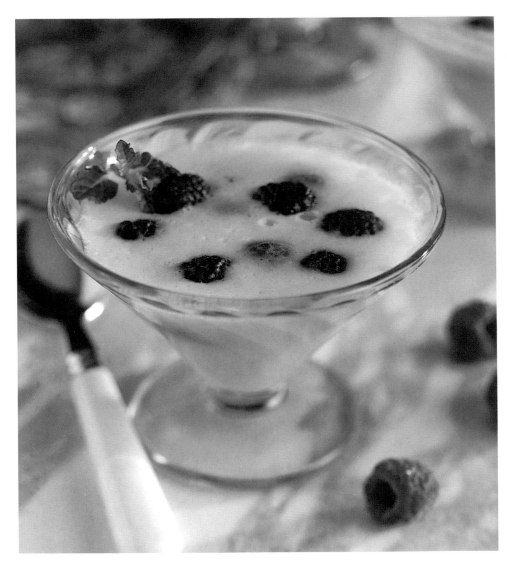

 Mango Mousse with Raspberry Speckles (page 54)

Disease Prevention—The Folic Acid Connection

• ***Heart Disease and Homocysteine.*** A growing body of research shows that high levels of homocysteine in the blood appears to be an independent risk factor for heart disease. This is similar to knowing that a high blood cholesterol level raises your risk for heart disease. While high blood cholesterol is related to eating too much saturated fat, a high homocysteine level is related to consuming inadequate B vitamins, particularly folic acid.

Three vitamins—folic acid, vitamin B_6, and vitamin B_{12}—are needed to help remove homocysteine from the blood. When there is a deficiency of one of these vitamins, homocysteine levels rise. Ironically, homocysteine levels have been measured in the past as a marker to indicate a deficiency of these vitamins. But of the trio, folic acid appears to be the key player.

Researchers began to see a correlation between high homocysteine levels and heart disease, but a recent international case-control study published in the *Journal of the American Medical Association* confirmed this relationship. This study, spanning nine countries, examined 750 people with vascular disease (which includes not only heart disease but strokes as well) and compared them to 800 people who had no disease. A striking independent risk of disease was found in patients who had high homocysteine levels.

The evidence is so strong that some researchers are recommending that homocysteine be measured when a patient is being evaluated for heart disease risk.

Many studies have demonstrated that folic acid reduces blood levels of homocysteine both in healthy volunteers and in those with moderately high levels of homocysteine. The optimal amount for keeping a healthy homocysteine level according to a recent study conducted at the University of Ulster, northern Ireland, is about 400 micrograms a day. That's about one cup of beans.

Another dietary key to preventing heart disease may very well be to eat a diet not only low in saturated fat but rich in folic acid.

• ***Depression—Can Beans Lift Your Spirits?*** It indeed appears that there is a relationship between depression and low levels of folic acid, but a cause and effect has yet to be demonstrated. Research is scanty but picking up in this area. Here's what we know so far:

- A substantial percentage of people with depression (15 to 38 percent) had low to deficient levels of folic acid in the blood, according to a review of several studies. Interestingly, most of these patients did not have any typical clinical symptoms of folic acid deficiency such as anemia or larger than normal-sized red blood cells (macrocytosis). Therefore, poor folate status would not show up on the usual blood measures, meaning that the folate level is low, but not severe enough to cause red blood cell damage.
- Compared to other people (either normal or with other mental diagnoses), depressed patients have been consistently found to have lower blood folic acid levels. Also patients with *very* low blood folate levels tend to have more severe ratings for depression.
- Several studies have also shown that patients with low folic acid levels tend to have poorer responses to antidepressant medication. Some researchers believe that supplemental folic acid may play a role in the treatment of depression.

What remains to be seen is whether folic acid deficiency causes depression or vice versa. For now it's the chicken-and-egg conundrum. For example, one symptom of depression is altered appetite. Low folic acid levels could merely be a marker for someone who has a diminished appetite triggered by depression. Or the subsequent low folic acid intake from a poor appetite might worsen an existing depression.

While the researchers have their work cut out, it certainly makes sense to make sure that you're getting enough folic acid in your diet.

NEURAL TUBE BIRTH DEFECTS

Each year in the United States approximately four thousand pregnancies are affected by spina bifida and anencephaly, the latter of which is fatal. Babies with spina bifida usually survive, but with serious physical deformity and mental retardation. Folic acid can reduce the occurrence of neural tube defects by at least 50 percent when consumed daily before conception and during early pregnancy. The neural tube is an organ present in the early stages of fetal development that becomes the brain and spinal cord.

In 1992 the Public Health Service (PHS) recommended that all women of childbearing age who are capable of becoming pregnant consume 400 micrograms of folic acid daily. Yet a 1996 Gallup poll survey commissioned by the March of Dimes found that only 15 percent of women surveyed were aware of the PHS recommendation. And many failed to get this amount of folic acid in the diet. Just one cup of dried beans will nearly meet this requirement, providing from 32 to 90 percent of the recommended amount of folic acid.

OTHER SOURCES OF FOLATE

I don't want to mislead you into thinking that beans are the only source of folic acid. There are certainly other sources, including green leafy vegetables, fortified breakfast cereals, and orange juice—but they pale in comparison to beans.

Five Ways to Sneak Beans into Meals

1. Sauces—when pureed, beans can make a fabulous sauce such as the one in the Enchilada Bake, page 130.

2. Surprise sneak—one of my best sneaks are the Dark Fudge Brownies, page 133, where black beans are pureed and incorporated into this delicious treat.

3. Souper soups—beans make a fabulous soup such as Lickety Split Pea Soup, page 126.

4. Dips—beans can make a great basis for a dip such as Red Pepper Hummus with Roasted Garlic, page 121.

5. Or serve them whole—sometimes all it takes is serving beans in a slightly different manner such as the Fiesta Black Bean Salad, page 132.

Beans: A Nutritional Powerhouse

One cup of cooked beans makes a significant contribution to folate, iron, fiber, and protein, meeting 30 percent or more of the recommended Daily Value.

	Folate micrograms	Iron milligrams	Fiber grams	Protein grams
Daily Value	**400**	**18**	**25**	**50**
Beans (1 cup, cooked):				
Black beans	256	3.6	15	15
Black-eyed peas	356	4.3	21	13
Chickpeas				
(garbanzo beans)	282	4.7	11	15
Kidney beans	229	5.2	15	15
Lentils	358	6.6	10	18
Lima beans	156	4.5	18	15
Navy beans	255	4.5	16	16
Pinto beans	294	4.5	20	14
Split peas	127	2.5	10	16
White beans,				
Great Northern	181	3.8	11	15

Source: Computer nutrition analysis using Food Processor v2.2 software

Twenty Ways to Increase Beans in Your Diet

1. Add kidney beans or garbanzo beans to your salad.
2. Order a bean burrito at a fast food restaurant.
3. Toss some pinto beans into a taco with the usual toppings.
4. Keep some canned beans in the pantry for a quick heat and eat lunch.
5. Take advantage of the instant bean soups in a cup; they are still plenty high in fiber.
6. When at a restaurant, order a bean-based soup for an appetizer.
7. Throw some beans into your favorite chili recipe.
8. Try a chili bean pita—fill a pita bread with your favorite chili beans, top with low-fat Cheddar cheese, and heat in the microwave until melted.
9. Try a new bean soup such as a lentil soup or pasta fagioli.
10. Try to make a pot of beans once a week. It's not only great for your budget but you can make several different types of meals, especially with pinto or black beans—from burritos to tostadas.
11. Make a double batch of split pea soup. Freeze the extra in individual bowls for tasty leftovers that get better with time.
12. Have the munchies? Buy your favorite low-fat bean dip and serve with toasted corn tortilla triangles for a tasty nacho snack.
13. Serve a side of baked beans with dinner.
14. Jazz up a low-fat hot dog with some chili beans.
15. Request "pot beans" or "charro beans" at Mexican restaurants. These beans are served whole without the added lard.
16. Many restaurants now offer a vegetarian chili (beans only)—give it a whirl.
17. Intimidated by cooking beans? Try an easy beginner's step and purchase the ready-to-make bean soups that come with an assortment of beans and seasonings. All you do is provide the water.
18. Try regional cuisine such as the popular southern dish, Hoppin' John. There are many twists to this dish, but all are rich in black-eyed peas.
19. At the food court in the mall, take a walk on the international side and try a Middle Eastern dish called falafel. It's a savory patty made from garbanzo beans tucked into a pita pocket and topped with tahini sauce.
20. For a very subtle bean cuisine, try the classic Italian soup, minestrone. The beans, though fewer than in traditional bean soups, soak up the rich tomato broth with a satisfying zest.

❎ Artichoke Hummus ❎

*This version of a popular Middle Eastern spread is a flavorful
way to eat beans. Tahini is like peanut butter, only made from sesame
seeds. It is usually sold in grocery stores with international
foods or in health food stores.*

THE SNEAK:

• Using a traditional recipe in which garbanzo beans are pureed and
jazzed up with marinated artichoke hearts

NUTRITION SCORECARD (PER SERVING)		NOTABLE NUTRIENT (PER SERVING)		
Calories	140			
Fat (grams)	4.7		AMOUNT	% DAILY VALUE
% Fat calories	29			
Protein (grams)	6	Fiber (grams)	6	24
Carbohydrates		Folic acid (micrograms)	128	32
(grams)	20			
Cholesterol				
(milligrams)	0			

1 (6-ounce) jar marinated artichoke hearts, do not drain	2 tablespoons lemon juice
	1 tablespoon tahini
	2 cloves garlic, minced
1 (15-ounce) can garbanzo beans, reserve 3 tablespoons of liquid	1 teaspoon Italian seasoning (or ½ teaspoon each basil and oregano)

In a food processor or blender add artichoke hearts with all of their liquid.
Puree until smooth. Drain the garbanzo beans, reserving 3 tablespoons
of the liquid; add to the artichoke puree. Add the lemon juice, tahini,
garlic, and Italian seasoning. Puree until smooth. Serve with pita bread or
raw vegetables.

Makes 7 servings ($^1/_4$ cup portion size) or 1$^3/_4$ cups

Red Pepper Hummus
❈ with Roasted Garlic ❈

This magnificent dip with its rich color is a real crowd pleaser. Don't be shocked that this recipe calls for an entire head of garlic—roasting mellows the flavor. Note how high the vitamin A level is, courtesy of the flavorful roasted peppers which are conveniently purchased in a jar.

THE SNEAK:

• Using a traditional recipe in which garbanzo beans are pureed and spiced up with red peppers and roasted garlic

NUTRITION SCORECARD (PER SERVING)		NOTABLE NUTRIENT (PER SERVING)		
Calories	153			
Fat (grams)	4.8		AMOUNT	% DAILY VALUE
% Fat calories	28			
Protein (grams)	6	Fiber (grams)	5	20
Carbohydrates		Vitamin A (RE)	956	96
(grams)	21	Folic acid (micrograms)	109	27
Cholesterol				
(milligrams)	0			

1 head garlic	2 tablespoons chopped sun-dried tomatoes, marinated in olive oil
1 tablespoon chicken broth	
½ teaspoon olive oil	
½ cup roasted red peppers (jar)	1 tablespoon lemon juice
1 (15-ounce) can garbanzo beans, reserve 3 tablespoons of the liquid	2 tablespoons tahini

Preheat the oven to 375°F. Cut ¼ inch off the top of the head of garlic, exposing the individual cloves. Put the garlic in a small baking dish with the chicken broth. Arrange the head, root end down. Drizzle the olive oil over the exposed cloves. Cover tightly with foil and bake for about 20 minutes. Remove the foil and roast until soft, 5 to 10 minutes more. Remove from the oven.

Using a toothpick remove the individual garlic cloves and add to a food processor or blender, along with the roasted red peppers. Puree until smooth. Add the garbanzo beans and the reserved 3 tablespoons of the liquid, chopped sun-dried tomatoes, lemon juice, and tahini. Puree until smooth.

Makes 7 servings ($1/4$ cup portion size) or $13/4$ cups

Bean Diet Lowers LDL

The same group of men was put on two different diets over a seven-week period. One diet was just a regular diet (the control) and the other was a bean diet in which four ounces of beans were substituted for foods having a similar nutrition profile (calories, fat, protein, and carbohydrate). The bean diet significantly decreased LDL (bad) cholesterol.
Journal of Lipid Research 38(6):1120–1128, 1997

Canned Beans Lower Cholesterol

Men with high blood cholesterol who ate canned pork and beans for three weeks lowered their cholesterol by 10 percent. That was a considerable accomplishment, since these volunteers were eating a high fat, high cholesterol diet at the time.
American Journal of Clinical Nutrition 51(6):1013–1019, 1990

Alphabet Soup

My neighbor Jim readily admits that he does not like beans. Yet he will eat beans pureed in this soup because he cannot see them! My kids love this soup because of the alphabet pasta. If you prefer a more sophisticated dish, orzo works equally well.

THE SNEAK:

• White beans are cooked, pureed, and added to the soup broth for a creamy texture.

NUTRITION SCORECARD (PER SERVING)		NOTABLE NUTRIENT (PER SERVING)		
Calories	279			
Fat (grams)	1.4		AMOUNT	% DAILY VALUE
% Fat calories	4			
Protein (grams)	14	Fiber (grams)	5	20
Carbohydrates		Vitamin A (RE)	713	71
(grams)	54	Folic acid (micrograms)	156	39
Cholesterol		Iron (milligrams)	4.7	31
(milligrams)	0			

1 cup chopped onions	1 (14½-ounce) can recipe-cut tomatoes (with liquid)
1 cup finely chopped carrots	1 teaspoon dried rosemary, crushed
4 cloves garlic, minced	1 teaspoon Italian seasoning or oregano
2 (14½-ounce) cans fat-free chicken broth	⅛ to ¼ teaspoon crushed red pepper
3 cups water	1 cup dry alphabet pasta
1 cup dried white beans, sorted and rinsed	

Add the onions, carrots, garlic, chicken broth, and water to a large 4-quart saucepan and bring to a boil. Add the beans, tomatoes, rosemary, Italian seasoning, and crushed red pepper. Bring to a boil again, then reduce the heat. Cover and simmer, stirring occasionally, for 1½ hours until the beans are tender.

Using a slotted spoon remove most of the beans and transfer to a blender or food processor. Blend or process until smooth. Return the mixture to the pan.

Stir in the alphabet pasta. Bring to a boil, then reduce the heat. Cover and simmer for about 8 minutes until the pasta is tender but firm.

Makes 6 main-dish servings (1 1/2 cups)

Beans Lower Cholesterol, Again

College students with high cholesterol levels fed a regular diet supplemented with a derivative of beans had a significantly lower cholesterol level. Another benefit was that HDL (good cholesterol) increased.
American Journal of Clinical Nutrition 66(6):1452–1460, 1997

✳ Black-eyed Pea Confetti Soup ✳

This inviting soup is a cinch to make and pleasing to the eyes—as if a merry party is taking place in your soup bowl.

THE SNEAK:

- Using canned beans makes this a very quick dish to prepare, especially for those who are intimidated by cooking dry beans from scratch.

NUTRITION SCORECARD (PER SERVING)		NOTABLE NUTRIENT (PER SERVING)		
Calories	151			
Fat (grams)	1.4		AMOUNT	% DAILY VALUE
% Fat calories	8			
Protein (grams)	9	Fiber (grams)	12	48
Carbohydrates		Folic acid (micrograms)	95	24
(grams)	27			
Cholesterol				
(milligrams)	0			

1	cup chopped onion	¼	teaspoon cumin
1	medium yellow bell pepper, chopped	⅛	teaspoon crushed red pepper
1	medium green bell pepper, chopped	2	(14½-ounce) cans fat-free chicken broth
2	cups finely snipped kale	2	(15-ounce) cans black-eyed peas, rinsed and drained
½	teaspoon chili powder		

Spray a large pot with nonstick vegetable spray. Add the onion and bell peppers; cook and stir over medium-high heat until the onion is translucent, about 5 minutes. Add the kale, chili powder, cumin, and crushed red pepper. Cook and stir until the kale is a vibrant green, about 2 minutes. Add the broth and black-eyed peas. Bring to a boil, reduce the heat, and simmer for 10 minutes. Remove from the heat.

Makes 6 servings (1 cup each)

Short-term Vitamin Deficiency Rapidly Raises Risk

According to one study, it takes only about thirty days for a diet low in folic acid to have a negative impact on homocysteine levels in the blood. (High levels of homocysteine have been blamed for increased risk of heart disease or stroke and may prove to be just as deadly as having high blood cholesterol.)
   USDA, AGS. *Food and Nutrition Research Briefs*, April 1, 1996

✳ Lickety Split Pea Soup ✳

I am surprised by the response of others when I mention split pea soup as one way to add beans to the diet. Typically most of my clients don't consider split peas in the bean category but are usually pleased to add this hearty dish to their menu repertoires.

The flat shape of the split pea allows for a quicker cooking time compared to other beans. Pair this up with some down-home corn bread for a wholesome and satisfying meal. Better yet, double the recipe and freeze one batch in individual bowls—you'll always have a home-cooked meal waiting for you.

THE SNEAK:

- Split peas are cooked and pureed into a soup—not exactly a sneak, but a nice and familiar way to use beans.

NUTRITION SCORECARD (PER SERVING)		NOTABLE NUTRIENT (PER SERVING)		
Calories	183			
Fat (grams)	0.6		AMOUNT	% DAILY VALUE
% Fat calories	3			
Protein (grams)	13	Fiber (grams)	8	32
Carbohydrates		Vitamin A (RE)	396	40
(grams)	33	Folic Acid (micrograms)	144	36
Cholesterol				
(milligrams)	0			

1	cup dry split peas, rinsed and sorted	1	large celery stalk, chopped
4	cups water	2	cloves garlic, minced
½	cup finely chopped carrot	1	bay leaf
½	cup finely chopped onion	½	teaspoon dried marjoram
		½	teaspoon salt

In a large saucepan combine the peas and water and bring to a boil. Reduce the heat and add the carrot, onion, celery, garlic, bay leaf, marjoram, and salt. Cover and simmer for 1 hour until tender, stirring occasionally. Discard the bay leaf. Puree the soup into two batches using a food processor, blender, or a portable hand blender and serve.

Makes 4 servings

My Favorite Pinto Beans

I am so fond of this versatile recipe that I usually make a double batch so I can easily make other meals using this base (the old principle of cook once but eat twice). Try serving this over brown rice, rolling it into a burrito, or using it in Tostadas Pronto Bar, page 128.

THE SNEAK:

- Using an old familiar staple of Mexican cuisine, mashed pinto beans

NUTRITION SCORECARD (PER SERVING)	
Calories	213
Fat (grams)	4.7
% Fat calories	19
Protein (grams)	16
Carbohydrates (grams)	28
Cholesterol (milligrams)	16

NOTABLE NUTRIENT (PER SERVING)	AMOUNT	% DAILY VALUE
Fiber (grams)	9	36
Folic Acid (micrograms)	195	49

1 cup dry pinto beans
1 (14½-ounce) can chicken broth
1½ cups water
⅛ teaspoon salt
1 (4-ounce) can diced green chili with liquid
½ cup (2 ounces) shredded reduced-fat Cheddar cheese
½ cup (2 ounces) shredded reduced-fat Jack cheese

In a large saucepan bring the beans, chicken broth, and water to a boil. Add the green chili with liquid, reduce the heat, and cover. Simmer for 1½ to 2 hours until the beans are tender. Using a portable hand blender or masher, puree or mash the beans until somewhat smooth yet lumpy.

Add the Cheddar and Jack cheeses and stir until melted and thoroughly combined.

Makes 5 servings (1/2 cup each)

Antioxidant Power

Pigments isolated from the bean seed coat of the common bean have been found to exhibit strong antioxidant activity; they may be a significant team player with the antioxidant vitamins C and E.

Journal of the American Dietetic Association 97(supplement 2):s199–s204, 1997

Tostadas Pronto Bar

Here's a quick meal that caters to personal preferences.

THE SNEAK:

- The mashed beans provide a subtle background against all of the tostada toppings.

NUTRITION SCORECARD (PER SERVING)	
Calories	213
Fat (grams)	4.7
% Fat calories	19
Protein (grams)	19
Carbohydrates (grams)	28
Cholesterol (milligrams)	16

NOTABLE NUTRIENT (PER SERVING)	AMOUNT	% DAILY VALUE
Fiber (grams)	14	56
Folic Acid (micrograms)	196	49

12 corn tortillas
1 batch My Favorite Pinto Beans (page 127)
3 cups chopped lettuce
2 chopped tomatoes
½ cup snipped cilantro
1 cup salsa

Preheat the oven to 400°F. Liberally spray 2 baking sheets with nonstick vegetable spray. Divide the tortillas between the baking sheets. Lightly spray the tortillas with nonstick spray. Bake for 10 to 12 minutes until light brown. Remove from the oven.

To assemble the tostadas: Spread about 3 tablespoons of beans over each tortilla. Place the remaining ingredients into serving bowls for each item. Let family members or friends top their tostadas with their favorite toppings—lettuce, tomatoes, cilantro, and salsa.

Makes 6 servings (2 tostadas each)

Beans Protect Against Colon Cancer

Colon cancer is lower in countries in which there is a high dry bean intake (especially Latin America) and is higher in countries such as the United States where dry bean consumption is low. A study examining fifteen countries with high dry bean intake showed a significantly lower rate of colon cancer.
Journal of Nutrition 127(12):2328–2333, 1997

✳ Enchilada Bake ✳

The first unsolicited words out of my toddler's mouth when he tried this were "mmmmm, tasty"—everyone in my family is a food critic! The tortillas are layered (lasagna style) rather than rolled individually, which is a nice little timesaving trick not to mention a lot less messy than the traditional rolled tortilla method.

THE SNEAK:

- Cooked lentils are pureed and incorporated into the enchilada sauce.

NUTRITION SCORECARD (PER SERVING)		NOTABLE NUTRIENT (PER SERVING)		
Calories	330			
Fat (grams)	10.3		AMOUNT	% DAILY VALUE
% Fat calories	26			
Protein (grams)	20	Fiber (grams)	7	28
Carbohydrates		Folic acid (micrograms)	117	29
(grams)	46	Calcium (milligrams)	282	28
Cholesterol		Iron (milligrams)	3.2	18
(milligrams)	20			

1	cup chopped onion	1	(10 ½-ounce) can fat-free condensed tomato soup	
¼	cup vinegar			
1	cup dry lentils, rinsed and sorted	1	teaspoon ground cumin	
2¾	cups water	12	corn tortillas	
1	green bell pepper, chopped	2	cups (8 ounces) shredded reduced-fat Cheddar cheese	
2	cloves garlic, minced			
1	(10-ounce) can enchilada sauce	½	cup sliced olives	
		⅓	cup chopped chives	

Combine the onion and vinegar in a small bowl, cover, and let stand until ready for assembling the enchiladas.

In a large saucepan combine the dry lentils, water, chopped bell pepper, and garlic. Bring to a boil. Reduce the heat and cover. Cook for 30 to 40 minutes until tender, stirring occasionally. Remove from the heat. Puree the lentils in a food processor or blender until smooth. Using the pan as your mixing bowl (why dirty a bowl), combine the pureed lentils, enchilada sauce, tomato soup, and cumin. Stir until smooth.

Preheat the oven to 350°F. Ladle a generous amount (about 1 cup) of lentil sauce to cover the bottom of a 9- × 13-inch pan. Place four of the corn tortillas on top of the sauce, tearing the tortillas to fit as needed. Add one third of the remaining sauce and spread evenly. Sprinkle one third of the marinated onion, cheese, and sliced olives. Repeat the layering, except before you place a layer of tortillas, "spackle" one side of the tortilla with sauce, placing the sauce side down toward the cheese. Add the sauce, onion, cheese, and olives. Repeat the layering. Cover the pan with foil and bake for 25 to 30 minutes until heated through and the cheese is almost melted. Remove the foil and bake for 5 additional minutes. Remove from the oven and sprinkle the chives on top of the enchilada. Let stand for 5 minutes before cutting.

Makes 8 servings

Folate-Rich Beans May Prevent Polyps

Colorectal cancer is the second leading cause of cancer deaths, claiming 60,000 lives each year. Each year, 150,000 new cases are diagnosed, and up to 90 percent are thought to be related to diet. People who eat high folate diets have fewer incidences of precancerous growths in the colon. Conversely, people with low folate diets have more of these polyps.
USDA, AGS. Food and Nutrition Research Briefs, July 1, 1996

Fiesta Black Bean Salad

This colorful salad is so delicious that I will often serve it as a main course (double the regular portions) with toasted corn tortillas adorned with melted low-fat cheese. This is also a great dish to take to a party because it's fast to prepare and can be made the night before.

THE SNEAK:

- The beans are surrounded with a colorful array of diced red and yellow peppers, scattered with green chives and cilantro.

NUTRITION SCORECARD (PER SERVING)		NOTABLE NUTRIENT (PER SERVING)	AMOUNT	% DAILY VALUE
Calories	148			
Fat (grams)	2.8			
% Fat calories	14			
Protein (grams)	7	Fiber (grams)	9	36
Carbohydrates (grams)	31	Vitamin C (milligrams)	83	138
Cholesterol (milligrams)	0			

- 2 tablespoons cider vinegar
- 1 tablespoon olive oil
- 3 cloves garlic, minced
- 2 ears yellow corn, husks and silks removed
- 2 (15-ounce) cans black beans
- 1 red bell pepper, finely diced
- 1 yellow bell pepper, finely diced
- ½ cup snipped chives (about ½ bunch)
- 3 tablespoons snipped cilantro
- 1 teaspoon ground cumin

In a small measuring cup whisk together the vinegar, olive oil, and garlic; set aside.

Wrap the corn in wax paper and microwave the ears together on high for 3 to 4 minutes. Allow to cool. Cut the kernels from the cobs using a sharp knife.

Place the beans in a colander and rinse and drain well.

In a large mixing bowl combine the corn kernels, rinsed black beans, red and yellow bell peppers, chives, cilantro, and cumin. Pour the garlic mixture over the black bean mixture and stir until well combined. Cover and chill for at least 1 hour. Serve cold.

Makes 6 servings (generous 1 cup each)

Beans Contain Anti-Cancer Ingredients

Rats fed a high bean diet had lower rates of colon cancer when compared to rats on a regular diet. Researchers concluded that dry beans are a rich source of phytochemicals and anti-cancer compounds.
Journal of Nutrition 127(12):2328–2333, 1997

✖ Dark Fudge Brownies ✖

Out of all my "sneaks," this is one of my favorites and has drawn rave reviews from my neighbors and family. Imagine their surprise when they learn the secret ingredient. One of these brownies has the same amount of fiber as a slice of whole wheat bread.

THE SNEAK:

- A can of black beans is pureed and incorporated into this delicious treat.
- Espresso powder intensifies the chocolate experience. Note: You can find espresso powder in most grocery stores, usually sold with instant coffee.

NUTRITION SCORECARD (PER SERVING)		NOTABLE NUTRIENT (PER SERVING)		
			AMOUNT	% DAILY VALUE
Calories	110			
Fat (grams)	3.4			
% Fat calories	26			
Protein (grams)	3	Fiber (grams)	2	8
Carbohydrates (grams)	19			
Cholesterol (milligrams)	1			

1	(15-ounce) can unseasoned black beans	2	cups sugar
4	ounces unsweetened chocolate	3	tablespoons all-purpose flour
1	tablespoon light butter	2	tablespoons instant espresso coffee powder
6	egg whites	½	cup chopped walnuts

Preheat the oven to 350°F. Spray a 9- × 13-inch pan with nonstick vegetable spray. Place the beans in a colander and rinse thoroughly under running water to remove "slime"; set aside and drain.

Place the chocolate and light butter in a small microwavable bowl. Microwave for 60 to 90 seconds, stirring every 30 seconds until smooth.

In a food processor or blender add the drained beans and 2 egg whites. Blend or process until smooth.

In a large bowl combine the bean puree, sugar, flour, espresso powder, and the remaining egg whites. With an electric mixer, beat until well combined. Mix in the melted chocolate.

Pour the brownie mixture into a prepared pan. Sprinkle the walnuts on top of the brownie batter. Bake for 30 to 35 minutes until the brownie pulls away from the sides of the pan.

Cool completely in the pan before cutting into bars—rows of six by five.

Makes 30 nice-sized brownies

Beans Are Blood Sugar Friendly

Of the starchy foods, beans generally have the least effect on blood sugar, which is why they are often promoted for dietary management of diabetes.
American Journal of Clinical Nutrition 66(6):1452–1460, 1997

Try These Other Bean Recipes

CHAPTER SIX

Fiber Imbiber

Whole Grains—Separating the Wheat from the Chaff

I was at the supermarket checkout stand when I realized that I forgot to buy bread. So I sent my ten-year-old daughter, Krystin, to get bread in aisle six. I started to get a bit worried because she was gone so long. Finally she came running up to me and said, "Sorry it took so long—I couldn't find any bread that listed *whole* wheat first on the ingredient list." My heart melted—I had mentioned this in passing to Krystin several weeks before. Not only did she remember how important whole grain is, she experienced a typical consumer conundrum of trying to find the true whole wheat bread.

You may think you are doing okay in the grain department, but if you are like most Americans, you'd better think again. A 1997 survey commissioned by the Wheat Foods Council found that while most Americans believe that they are eating enough grain servings (six to eleven servings according to the Food Guide Pyramid), only 12 percent met the minimum recommendation of six servings.

How important whole grains are in their contribution to fiber in our diet becomes very apparent when you consider that on a per serving basis, most fruits and vegetables contain less than two grams of fiber and most refined grains contain less than one gram. Only beans, *whole grains, and concentrated grain products typically have more fiber* than fruits and vegetables. Which leads us to the purpose of this chapter— why fiber is so important and how to get more whole grains into your diet.

Mighty, Mighty Fiber

There are hundreds of studies that attest to the health benefits of fiber, from preventing chronic diseases such as diabetes, heart disease, and cancer to weight loss. Let's take a closer look.

• *Heart Disease*—There is no doubt that high fiber diets reduce the risk of heart disease. Three types of grain fibers in particular have been found to lower cholesterol: oats, barley, and rice bran. These grains contain a compound called tocotrienol that is a potent off switch that prevents the body from making cholesterol. (Most of the cholesterol found in your blood is made by the body, not supplied by the diet.) Some studies have shown that there may also be some other benefits that fiber confers on heart health beyond lowering blood cholesterol levels. In fact, a twelve-year prospective study reported that just a six gram increase in dietary fiber was associated with a 25 percent reduction in death from coronary heart disease independent of any other factors in the diet.

• *Cancer*—High fiber diets reduce the risk of developing many types of cancer, but in particular colorectal cancer. One particular meta study analyzed the results from sixty different studies on diet and colon cancer and found that fiber was highly protective against colorectal cancer. In fact, when all the data from the sixty studies was pooled, researchers found that the highest fiber eaters had only half the chance of developing cancer as the lowest fiber group.

• *Weight Loss*—While there is not a study that shows a clear link between obesity and fiber intake, there are some compelling studies that show:

• *The greater the fiber intake at mealtime, the fewer the calories you absorb from that meal.* (And if you don't absorb a calorie it can't contribute to your fat stores.) Researchers estimate that if men doubled their daily fiber intake from the U.S. average of 18 grams to 36 grams (the highest amount of fiber used in the study), they would absorb 130 fewer calories per day. Similarly, if women doubled their fiber intake from 12 to 24 grams per day, they would have 90 fewer calories to worry about.

• High fiber foods take longer to eat, which increases the feeling of satiety and may therefore result in eating less food.

• *Higher fiber breakfasts resulted in less lunch eaten.* Volunteers at the University of Minnesota were fed a high fiber breakfast (22 grams of fiber) for five days and then monitored. The results—they ate less at lunch. While this is a very short-term study, on a long-term basis this may have a significant impact on weight.

• *Diabetes*—Fiber plays a role in preventing and treating diabetes because it slows the rate at which glucose enters the bloodstream. Since 1976 research has documented the benefits of high fiber diets for diabetics. In a mega study analyzing fifty-three different studies on diabetes and fiber, nearly two thirds reported that high fiber diets improved blood sugar control, not to mention an improvement in cholesterol, a common problem in diabetics. No wonder that diabetes is more prevalent in people with low fiber diets than in those with high fiber diets.

• *Diverticulitis*—It's no secret that a high fiber diet is key to keeping food traveling smoothly and regularly throughout the intestinal tract. Conversely, when people eat a low fiber diet, they have a very low-bulk stool that causes difficulties with elimination. In some cases people develop abnormal pouches in the intestinal tract called diverticulosis, which affects about one out of three people in North America. Imagine squeezing a long balloon like the ones used to mold animal shapes at the circus. When pressure is applied, the balloon bulges out—like the pouch that develops in the intestine on a low fiber diet. Once these pouches are formed, food particles can get trapped there, resulting in the painful inflammation called diverticulitis.

All Fibers Are Not Created Equal

The benefits of fiber alone make it easy to get swept up on the fiber bandwagon; while not a bad thing, it's important to note that getting a *variety* of fiber is very important. This is because there are two different types of fiber that impart different health benefits, both of which are considerable.

Let's start with the basics. Fiber is the nondigestible part of plants, that is, fruits, vegetables, and grains. Our bodies do not possess the necessary enzyme to break down fiber. Therefore, fiber remains too big to pass into our bloodstream from the digestive tract and literally moves through us.

Soluble versus insoluble. There are two types of fiber, insoluble and soluble. While neither of these fibers is absorbed by the body, they do behave differently in water. Soluble fiber absorbs water, forming a gellike substance. You have probably seen this in action when you have added water (or milk) to oatmeal, which is a soluble fiber—it swells in the bowl, especially as it cools. Benefits of soluble fiber in particular include lowering blood cholesterol and moderating blood sugar levels.

Insoluble fiber such as wheat bran does not absorb water and passes through our digestive system in more or less its original form. Benefits of this type of fiber are conferred upon intestinal health, including the prevention of colorectal cancer, hemorrhoids, and constipation.

How Much Fiber Is Enough?

Adults. For adults the recommended amount of fiber is 25 to 35 grams of fiber each day. Or 10 to 13 grams of fiber for each 1,000 calories in your diet. Unfortunately, most Americans fall very short, averaging only 12 to 18 grams of fiber daily.

Children. There's an easy way to figure children's fiber needs by using the Age Plus Five formula, and you won't need a calculator. Take the age of the child and add five. That simple formula equals the daily amount of fiber (grams) a child from age three to eighteen should eat daily. For example, a ten-year-old child needs to aim for 15 grams of fiber (10 + 5 = 15).

Most fruits and vegetables contain less than 2 grams of fiber per serving, which means you'll get about 10 grams of fiber from fruits and vegetables if you hit the minimum quota of five servings each day (combined from each group). Refined whole grain products contain less than 1 gram of fiber per serving. So even if you get the minimum six grain servings a day (as recommended in the Food Guide Pyramid), without focusing on the whole grain quality, that's only another six grams of fiber.

You can see how it's all too easy for the average American to fall short on fiber.

WHAT IS A WHOLE GRAIN?

Now here's the rub—you may think you are eating a whole grain, but it may not be so! For example, bread made with "wheat flour" or "unbleached wheat flour" is not a whole grain bread. Wheat flour is merely white flour! Since white flour is made from wheat, it can be listed on the food label as wheat flour—go figure. The critical term to look for is the adjective "whole" in the ingredient list on the food label as in *whole* wheat flour. Other terms that are just as misleading (especially on bread, crackers, and cereal boxes) are "multi-grain" and "whole grain goodness." These terms are meaningless—there may be a smidgen of whole grain, but unless you see whole grain or whole wheat as the first ingredient, you basically have a white flour product.

When it comes to cereals, keep in mind that Cream of Wheat and Cream of Rice are not whole grain cereals. Similarly, couscous and regular pasta are not whole grains; they are made from refined wheat flour.

Here are some specific examples of whole grains: whole wheat flour, brown rice, oatmeal, oats, wheat germ, barley, millet, and quinoa.

Use the Food Label to Your Advantage. Use the nutrition facts label to get the scoop on the fiber content. Use the Percent Daily Value (%DV) for a quick reference:

• 20 percent DV or higher is considered an excellent or high source of fiber. It means that you are getting at least 5 grams of fiber per serving.

• 10 to 19 percent DV is considered a good source of fiber. It means that you will be getting at least 2.5 grams of fiber per serving.

NUTRITIONAL BENEFITS OF WHOLE GRAINS

While whole grains are loaded with fiber, it's just as important that they contain significantly more nutrients than their refined counterparts. When whole grain is refined, many of the nutrients are stripped away and you are left with a nutritionally inferior product. Look at the chart comparing whole wheat flour and white flour on page 141. Whole wheat flour has ten times the vitamin E content, six times the magnesium, and two to four times the selenium, potassium, and zinc. What a difference!

It's also important to point out that this nutrient difference may also have a hidden impact on the many fiber studies demonstrating health benefits. Most fiber studies are based on people eating real foods, and it may very well be that the way fiber is packaged (whole food, courtesy of Mother Nature) offers the real benefit, not just the fiber itself. So if you were thinking of adding a couple of fiber supplements to your morning routine, you may still be missing out.

A LITTLE WORD ABOUT CARBOHYDRATES, GRAINS, AND WEIGHT

Carbohydrates are not inherently fattening, although that seems to be the prevailing belief of many Americans. While 72 percent of consumers surveyed agreed that "complex carbohydrates" are good for you, almost 40 percent thought that "starches" such as bread and pasta should be avoided and are particularly fattening. It just isn't so.

Five Ways to Sneak Whole Grains into Meals

1. Instead of rice—anywhere rice goes a whole grain will be an excellent ingredient such as Chicken Bundles with Apricot Stuffing and Honey-Orange Sauce, page 161.

2. Bake it—when baking, use part whole wheat flour, such as Jeff's Thick-Crust Bread-Machine Pizza, page 151, or Cinnayum Rolls, page 165.

3. Beyond whole wheat—explore other grains such as barley. See Barley Soup, page 144.

4. Crunchy toppings and coatings—use whole grains for toppings and coatings such as Crunchy Oven-Fried Chicken, page 152, or Apple-Pear Crisp, page 146.

5. Extra stealthy—the Streusel Coffee Cake, page 163, is a good example of where a whole grain is used and no one would even know it.

Whole Wheat Flour Versus White Flour

Compare the nutritional difference between whole wheat and white flour—
it's more than just the fiber.

	Whole Wheat	White
Fiber (grams)	13.9	4.1
Vitamin E (mg)	3.1	0.3
Magnesium (mg)	166	28
Selenium (mcg)	85	42
Potassium (mg)	486	134
Zinc (mg)	3.5	0.9

Source: Computer nutrition analysis using Food Processor v2.2 software

Twenty Ways to Increase Fiber in Your Diet

1. Buy bread that uses whole grain as the first ingredient, particularly whole wheat flour.
2. Use brown rice instead of white rice—even instant brown rice is an improvement in the fiber department.
3. When baking breads, cookies, muffins, or brownies, try using one third to one half whole wheat flour in place of all-purpose flour.
4. Buy whole grain crackers—be sure that the first ingredient is whole wheat flour or a type of whole grain.
5. When eating out, request that sandwiches be made on whole wheat bread.
6. Serve whole wheat breadsticks with soup or salad.
7. Choose a whole grain cereal that provides at least 5 grams of fiber or more per serving.
8. Use whole wheat tortillas when making burritos or quesadillas.
9. Add wild rice to your favorite rice dish—it's a whole grain.
10. Throw a little wheat germ or oat bran into your favorite cobbler topping.
11. Use a whole wheat hamburger bun when making hamburgers or sloppy joes.
12. Try whole wheat pastry flour as a nice introduction to using whole wheat flour. It has a much finer texture and is lighter in color.
13. For a convenient breakfast, buy frozen whole grain waffles—just pop into the toaster.
14. Stuff a whole wheat pita bread with your favorite sandwich fixings.
15. Enrich your regular breakfast cereal by tossing in some wheat germ, wheat bran, or oat bran.
16. Crumble graham crackers with wheat germ and cinnamon. Sprinkle over applesauce for an afternoon snack.
17. Top a whole wheat pita bread with pizza sauce, mozzarella cheese, and a dash of oregano. Heat in the microwave until melted for a quick pita pizza snack.
18. Experiment with new grains. Try quinoa or millet as a side dish instead of rice.
19. When eating out for breakfast, try buckwheat pancakes.
20. Munch on popcorn (low fat, please) for a satisfying whole grain snack.

Fiber Content of Grains

GRAIN	FIBER (grams)
Amaranth, ½ cup dry	14.8
Barley, whole, ½ cup dry	15.9
Barley, pearled, ½ cup dry	13.7
Bread, white, 1-ounce slice	0.5
Bread, whole wheat, 1-ounce slice	2.1
Bulgur wheat, ½ cup dry	12.8
Flour, all-purpose (white), ½ cup	2.0
Flour, whole wheat, ½ cup	6.9
Oat bran, ½ cup dry	7.3
Pita bread, white, 1	1.3
Pita bread, whole wheat, 1	3.2
Quinoa, ½ cup dry	5
Rice, brown (medium grain), ½ cup cooked	1.7
Rice, white (medium grain), ½ cup cooked	0.3
Rice, wild, ½ cup cooked	1.0
Rolled oats, ½ cup dry	4.1
Wheat bran, ½ cup dry	12.6
Wheat germ, ½ cup dry	8.1

✄ Barley Soup ✄

Barley adds a wonderful texture to this satisfying soup. To make this soup a little quicker I chop all my vegetables (except the tomato) in the food processor, but a good knife will certainly do.

THE SNEAK:

- Barley is the key ingredient for fiber, yet it is such a natural component of a hearty soup that it fits right in without screaming fiber.

NUTRITION SCORECARD (PER SERVING)		NOTABLE NUTRIENT (PER SERVING)		
Calories	134			
Fat (grams)	1.0		AMOUNT	% DAILY VALUE
% Fat calories	7			
Protein (grams)	6	Fiber (grams)	6	24
Carbohydrates (grams)	26			
Cholesterol (milligrams)	1			

1	cup sliced mushrooms	2	teaspoons dried thyme
2	medium carrots, finely chopped	1	tomato, diced
2	stalks celery, chopped	4	cups beef broth
1	medium onion, chopped	⅓	cup fresh parsley
½	cup pearl barley, rinsed		

Spray a 4-quart pan with nonstick vegetable spray. Add the mushrooms, carrots, celery, onion, barley, and thyme. Cook and stir until the vegetables are tender, about 10 minutes.

Add the tomato and beef broth to the pot. Bring the soup to a boil, stirring frequently. Reduce the heat to medium and simmer until the barley is tender and the soup is beginning to thicken, about 45 minutes. Stir in the parsley and serve.

Makes 4 servings (1 cup each)

Silver Dollar Pancakes with Rowdy Raspberry Sauce

My niece, who is not so fond of whole wheat foods, pronounced these the best pancakes ever. What's particularly nice about this recipe is that the ingredients are usually on hand, which is why I often serve this to house guests for breakfast.

THE SNEAK:

- The secret is in the sauce. The warm raspberry sauce crowns the pancakes in a cheerful display and helps keep the pancakes tender. The cinnamon in the pancakes also adds a nice background flavor.

NUTRITION SCORECARD (PER SERVING)	
Calories	354
Fat (grams)	0.8
% Fat calories	2
Protein (grams)	11
Carbohydrates (grams)	79
Cholesterol (milligrams)	2

NOTABLE NUTRIENT (PER SERVING)	AMOUNT	% DAILY VALUE
Fiber (grams)	8	32

RASPBERRY SAUCE

1 (12-ounce) bag frozen raspberries (do not thaw)
1/3 cup sugar
1 teaspoon cornstarch

PANCAKES

1 cup nonfat vanilla yogurt
1 teaspoon baking soda
3 egg whites, lightly beaten
1/4 cup skim milk
1 cup whole wheat flour
1 tablespoon sugar
1 1/2 teaspoons cinnamon

To make the sauce: In a small saucepan combine the raspberries and sugar. Cook and stir occasionally over medium heat. As the raspberries cook they will liquefy. Remove about 2 teaspoons of the raspberry liquid and combine with the cornstarch until smooth. Add the cornstarch mixture to the raspberries. Cook and stir until bubbly. Cover and remove from the heat.

To make the pancakes: In a large bowl whisk together the yogurt and baking soda. Whisk in the egg whites and skim milk. Add the whole wheat flour, sugar, and cinnamon and stir until just moistened.

Spray an unheated griddle or large skillet with nonstick vegetable spray. Heat the griddle over medium heat. For each pancake, pour a scant tablespoonful onto the hot griddle. Cook until the pancakes are bubbly and slightly dry around the edges. Using a spatula, turn over and cook until golden brown.

Serve the pancakes with a generous dollop of raspberry sauce.

Makes 4 servings (36 silver dollar pancakes)

❈ Apple-Pear Crisp ❈

While I used pears to help boost the fiber level, they add a complementary sweetness and texture. This is one of my favorite recipes and it's so satisfying to know that each serving provides 5 grams of fiber (more than a bowl of oatmeal!).

THE SNEAK:

- Fiber is boosted by using pears for some of the apples. Pears have nearly twice the fiber.
- The crisp topping is a combination of oats and wheat germ, which is pulsed to a crumbly texture that allows the presence of wheat germ to be discreet.

NUTRITION SCORECARD (PER SERVING)		NOTABLE NUTRIENT (PER SERVING)		
Calories	278			
Fat (grams)	5.2		AMOUNT	% DAILY VALUE
% Fat calories	16			
Protein (grams)	3	Fiber (grams)	5	20
Carbohydrates (grams)	58			
Cholesterol (milligrams)	10			

FRUIT FILLING

- 3 medium apples (1 pound), peeled and thinly sliced
- 3 medium pears (1 pound), peeled and thinly sliced
- ¼ cup sugar
- 1 teaspoon cinnamon
- ½ teaspoon nutmeg

CRISP TOPPING

- ½ cup brown sugar
- ⅓ cup oats
- ¼ cup wheat germ
- ¼ cup all-purpose flour
- 1 teaspoon cinnamon
- ½ teaspoon nutmeg
- ¼ cup well-chilled light butter

Preheat the oven to 375°F. Lightly coat a shallow 8- × 8-inch baking dish or 9 inch pie plate with nonstick cooking spray.

In a large bowl combine the apples, pears, sugar, cinnamon, and nutmeg. Toss until lightly coated. Transfer to a prepared baking dish.

In a food processor or blender add the brown sugar, oats, wheat germ, flour, cinnamon, and nutmeg. Pulse until thoroughly mixed. Using a cheese grater, shred the chilled butter and add to the brown sugar mixture. Pulse until crumbly.

Sprinkle the topping over the apple mixture. Bake for 40 to 45 minutes until the fruit is tender and the filling is bubbly. Serve warm.

Makes 6 servings

✕ Date Nut Bran Muffins ✕

This moist muffin has an inviting accent of cinnamon and orange peel. It's a great on-the-run breakfast packed with nutrients, especially vitamin A and fiber.

THE SNEAK:

- An interesting texture contrast—a moist muffin contributed by the baby food carrots. Nuts and dates add a delightful chewiness.

NUTRITION SCORECARD (PER SERVING)		NOTABLE NUTRIENT (PER SERVING)		
Calories	274			
Fat (grams)	5.1		AMOUNT	% DAILY VALUE
% Fat calories	15			
Protein (grams)	8	Fiber (grams)	6.5	26
Carbohydrates		Vitamin A (RE)	565	56
(grams)	57			
Cholesterol				
(milligrams)	2			

1	cup 100% bran cereal (such as Kellogg's All-Bran)	2	egg whites, lightly beaten
1	cup buttermilk	⅓	cup honey
⅔	cup all-purpose flour	1	(4-ounce) jar baby food carrots
⅓	cup whole wheat flour	⅓	cup chopped dates
¼	cup sugar	⅓	cup chopped walnuts
1	teaspoon baking soda	2	teaspoons finely shredded orange peel (zest)
1	teaspoon cinnamon		

In a large mixing bowl combine the cereal and buttermilk. Let stand for about 10 minutes until the cereal softens. Meanwhile, spray six large 3-inch muffin pan cups with nonstick vegetable spray. Preheat the oven to 375°F.

In a small bowl combine the all-purpose flour, whole wheat flour, sugar, baking soda, and cinnamon.

Add the egg whites, honey, and carrots to the cereal mixture. Beat well. Add the flour mixture, stirring just until moistened. Fold in the dates, walnuts, and orange peel.

Spoon the batter into the prepared muffin cups, filling each ¾ full. Bake for 20 to 22 minutes until a toothpick inserted in the center comes out clean. Cool the muffins in the muffin cups for 5 minutes. Then remove and serve warm.

Makes 6 large muffins

Increasing Fiber Decreases Colorectal Cancer Risk

It is estimated that the risk of colorectal cancer could be reduced by about one third in the United States if fiber intake from food sources were increased by an average of 13 grams per day.
Journal of the American Dietetic Association 97(10):1157–1159, 1997

Whole Grains Are Rich in Phytochemicals

Refining wheat causes about a 200- to 300-fold loss in phytochemicals—nature's health-enhancing compounds.
Journal of the American Dietetic Association 97(suppl 2):s119–s204, 1997

❋ Wild Rice Pilaf ❋

Wild rice adds a special touch to rice dishes. Besides imparting a nutty flavor, it's also naturally high in fiber. Note: If you prefer a stickier texture use a short grain brown rice.

THE SNEAK:

• Adding wild rice and other goodies to brown rice

NUTRITION SCORECARD (PER SERVING)		NOTABLE NUTRIENT (PER SERVING)		
Calories	191			
Fat (grams)	1.8		AMOUNT	% DAILY VALUE
% Fat calories	9			
Protein (grams)	7	Fiber (grams)	2.5	10
Carbohydrates (grams)	37			
Cholesterol (milligrams)	0			

½ cup chopped onion
½ cup sliced mushrooms
¼ cup chopped celery
1 clove garlic, minced

⅔ cup medium grain brown rice
⅓ cup wild rice
2 cups chicken broth

Spray a saucepan with nonstick vegetable spray. Cook and stir the onion, mushrooms, celery, garlic, brown rice, and wild rice until the vegetables are tender. Stir in the chicken broth. Bring to a boil and reduce the heat. Cover and simmer for about 45 minutes until the rice is tender and the liquid is absorbed.

Makes 4 servings

Jeff's Thick-Crust Bread-Machine Pizza

For years my husband, Jeff, wanted a bread machine. When I realized he wasn't joking I bought him one for his birthday, and am I sorry we didn't get it sooner. *It gets used at least once a week to make pizza and Jeff has turned into the best pizza maker ever. But when cooking Jeff does not measure; he prefers the eyeball technique (which he's quite good at). Therefore, to capture the right flavor and texture I measured each ingredient* after *Jeff threw it into the bread machine—a bit tedious, but worth it!*

THE SNEAK:

- Incorporating whole wheat flour into the pizza dough

NUTRITION SCORECARD (PER SERVING—2 SLICES)		NOTABLE NUTRIENT (PER SERVING—2 SLICES)	AMOUNT	% DAILY VALUE
Calories	482			
Fat (grams)	10.4			
% Fat calories	19			
Protein (grams)	22	Fiber (grams)	6.5	26
Carbohydrates (grams)	76	Calcium (milligrams)	295	30
Cholesterol (milligrams)	24			

DOUGH

- 1 cup water
- 2 teaspoons canola oil
- 2 cups all-purpose bread-machine flour
- 1 cup whole wheat flour
- 1 tablespoon sugar
- 2 teaspoons bread-machine yeast
- 3/4 teaspoon Italian seasoning or oregano
- 1/4 teaspoon salt

TOPPING

- 1/2 cup pizza sauce
- 1 1/2 cups mozzarella cheese

To make the dough: Add the water, oil, bread-machine flour, whole wheat flour, sugar, yeast, Italian seasoning, and salt to the bread machine. Select the dough setting and operate according to manufacturer's directions.

Spray a 12-inch round pizza pan with nonstick vegetable spray. Lightly flour your fingertips. Remove the dough and flatten it into a disc and place it on the pizza pan. Gently stretch the dough working it to fit the pizza pan. Build up the edges slightly. Do not let rise. Bake in a 425°F oven for about 8 minutes until lightly browned. Reduce the oven to 325°F and remove pizza crust.

Spread the pizza sauce over the hot crust and sprinkle with the cheese. Bake for 10 to 15 minutes until bubbly.

VARIATION: Top with Italian Salsa (page 34) or your favorite vegetables.

Makes 4 servings, 8 slices

Crunchy Oven-Fried Chicken

I love making this particular recipe with drumsticks because they are much easier to eat with their built-in handles, making them a natural for a picnic. Tip: To prevent your hands from getting gooey, use one hand for "dry-dipping" and the other for "wet-dipping."

THE SNEAK:

- Wheat germ and wheat bran are incorporated into the crispy coating.

NUTRITION SCORECARD (PER SERVING—3 DRUMSTICKS)	
Calories	322
Fat (grams)	8.8
% Fat calories	25
Protein (grams)	4
Carbohydrates (grams)	16
Cholesterol (milligrams)	123

NOTABLE NUTRIENT (PER SERVING—3 DRUMSTICKS)	AMOUNT	% DAILY VALUE
Fiber (grams)	3	12
Iron (milligrams)	3.9	22

½	cup crushed cornflake crumbs	⅛	teaspoon black pepper
⅓	cup wheat germ	¼	cup all-purpose flour
3	tablespoons unprocessed	2	egg whites, lightly beaten
	wheat bran	12	chicken drumsticks, skin
1½	teaspoons paprika		removed
¼	teaspoon salt		

Preheat the oven to 375°F. Lightly spray a cookie sheet with nonstick vegetable spray and set aside.

In a shallow bowl combine the cornflake crumbs, wheat germ, bran, paprika, salt, and pepper.

Place the flour in another shallow bowl or plate. And put the egg whites in a separate bowl.

To coat the chicken: First roll the drumsticks in the flour to evenly cover all sides. Then dip the chicken in the egg whites and roll in the cornflake crumb mixture. Bake for 35 to 40 minutes until no longer pink and juices run clear.

Makes 4 servings (3 drumsticks each)

Refined Flour Products on the Rise

Among the fastest growing "grain" foods in this country are refined flour products (not whole grains), including pasta, pizza crust, pretzels, and bagels.
The State of America's Plate, Wheat Foods Council: Englewood, CO, 1997

❊ Herbed Biscuits ❊

While these savory biscuits call for four specific fresh herbs, feel free to use any herb combination as long as they are fresh.

THE SNEAK:

- The fresh herbs serve two stealthy purposes: They add flavor and color to break up the brownness of the biscuit.
- The crowning Parmesan cheese puts a flavorful disguise on top of the biscuit.

NUTRITION SCORECARD (PER SERVING—1 BISCUIT)		NOTABLE NUTRIENT (PER SERVING—1 BISCUIT)		
Calories	154			
Fat (grams)	4.1		AMOUNT	% DAILY VALUE
% Fat calories	23			
Protein (grams)	6	Fiber (grams)	3	12
Carbohydrates				
(grams)	25			
Cholesterol				
(milligrams)	10			

1½ cups whole wheat flour
1 cup all-purpose flour
4 teaspoons baking powder
2 teaspoons sugar
¼ teaspoon salt
¼ cup chilled stick light butter
¾ cup buttermilk
1 tablespoon chopped fresh basil

1 tablespoon chopped fresh rosemary
1 tablespoon chopped fresh parsley
1 tablespoon chopped fresh dill
3 tablespoons grated Parmesan cheese

Preheat the oven to 450°F. Combine the whole wheat flour, all-purpose flour, baking powder, sugar, and salt. Using a cheese grater, shred the chilled butter. Using a pastry cutter or your fingertips, cut in the shredded butter until the mixture forms coarse crumbs. Add the buttermilk and herbs and stir until the mixture forms a ball. Gently knead the dough on a lightly floured surface for 10 to 12 strokes. Roll the dough out on a lightly floured surface to ½-inch thickness. Using a 3-inch round cutter, cut out the biscuits. Transfer the biscuits to a baking sheet. Lightly press about 1 teaspoon Parmesan cheese on top of each biscuit. Bake for 10 to 12 minutes until golden.

Makes 8 biscuits

High Fiber, No Pain

Men who ate an average of 32 grams of fiber each day were 42 percent less likely to report symptoms of diverticular disease (painful inflammation of the intestine) than men who averaged 13 grams a day.
Nutrition Action Health Letter 24(2):1–11, 1997

✿ Oriental Barley Salad ✿

The combination of a chewy texture with a subtle Asian flavor makes this salad a winner.

THE SNEAK:

• The cooked barley resembles a rice salad, yet it offers so much more fiber.

NUTRITION SCORECARD (PER SERVING)		NOTABLE NUTRIENT (PER SERVING)		
Calories	151			
Fat (grams)	2.8		AMOUNT	% DAILY VALUE
% Fat calories	16			
Protein (grams)	3	Fiber (grams)	5	20
Carbohydrates (grams)	28			
Cholesterol (milligrams)	0			

1½ cups fat-free chicken broth
1 cup pearl barley
½ cup finely diced red bell pepper
¼ cup snipped cilantro

2 tablespoons seasoned rice vinegar
2 tablespoons pineapple juice
1 tablespoon dark sesame oil
1 clove garlic, minced
⅛ teaspoon crushed red pepper

In a medium saucepan combine the chicken broth and barley. Bring to a boil and reduce the heat. Cover and simmer for 12 to 15 minutes until the liquid is absorbed.

In a mixing bowl combine the barley, bell pepper, and cilantro.

To make the dressing: In a small bowl whisk together the vinegar, pineapple juice, sesame oil, garlic, and crushed red pepper. Pour the dressing over the barley mixture. Toss to coat. Cover and chill for at least 1 hour.

Makes 6 side-dish servings (½ cup each)

Tabbouleh Salad

This classic salad is naturally high in fiber because of its cracked wheat (bulgur) content.

THE SNEAK:

- Sometimes, the best sneak is to serve a traditional food that already uses a particular healthful ingredient. In this case, it's wholesome cracked wheat.

NUTRITION SCORECARD (PER SERVING)		NOTABLE NUTRIENT (PER SERVING)	AMOUNT	% DAILY VALUE
Calories	107	Fiber (grams)	5	20
Fat (grams)	3.2	Vitamin C (milligrams)	19	31
% Fat calories	24			
Protein (grams)	3			
Carbohydrates (grams)	19			
Cholesterol (milligrams)	0			

- 1 cup bulgur (cracked wheat)
- 1 cup boiling chicken broth
- 3 tomatoes, chopped
- 1 medium cucumber, finely diced
- ½ cup snipped parsley
- ⅓ cup finely diced red onion
- 3 tablespoons snipped fresh mint
- ⅓ cup fresh lemon juice
- 3 tablespoons chicken broth
- 4 teaspoons olive oil
- 2 cloves garlic, minced
- ⅛ teaspoon salt

In a large bowl stir together the bulgur and broth. Let stand for about 15 minutes until the water is absorbed. Stir in the tomatoes, cucumber, parsley, red onions, and mint.

In a small bowl stir together the lemon juice, chicken broth, olive oil, garlic, and salt. Add the lemon juice mixture to the bulgur. Gently stir until combined. Cover and refrigerate for at least 2 hours.

Makes 8 servings (¾ cup each)

✳ Figgy Date Bars ✳

*The date and fig filling is sandwiched between a cookie crumb mixture,
a most tasty way to bolster your fiber intake any time of the day.*

THE SNEAK:

- A retinue of high fiber ingredients: oats, whole wheat flour, wheat
  germ, dates, and figs

NUTRITION SCORECARD (PER SERVING)		NOTABLE NUTRIENT (PER SERVING)		
Calories	187			
Fat (grams)	5.3		AMOUNT	% DAILY VALUE
% Fat calories	24			
Protein (grams)	3	Fiber (grams)	4	16
Carbohydrates (grams)	40			
Cholesterol (milligrams)	8			

FILLING

1	cup chopped dates
12	dried figs, finely chopped
½	cup water
½	teaspoon grated lemon peel
1	teaspoon vanilla extract

CRUST AND TOPPING

⅔	cup rolled oats
½	cup wheat germ
½	cup brown sugar
⅓	cup whole wheat flour
¼	cup chopped walnuts
1	teaspoon cinnamon
6	tablespoons chilled light butter

To make the filling: Combine the dates, figs, water, and lemon peel in a
medium saucepan. Heat to boiling. Reduce heat and cover. Cook and occasionally stir until the dates are tender and the water is absorbed, about
5 minutes. Remove from the heat and stir in the vanilla.

Preheat the oven to 350°F. Lightly spray an 8-inch square baking pan
with nonstick vegetable spray.

To make the crust and topping: In a food processor add the oats,
wheat germ, brown sugar, whole wheat flour, chopped walnuts, and
cinnamon. Pulse until ingredients are thoroughly combined. Grate

the chilled light butter and add to the oat mixture. Pulse until crumbly.

To assemble: Sprinkle half of the oat mixture into the prepared pan and press into a thin, even layer. (I like to do this by putting my hand in a small plastic bag—the crumbs do not stick.) Drop spoonfuls of the filling evenly over the crust. Gently spread on a thin layer with a small flexible spatula. Sprinkle the remaining crust mixture evenly over the top; press down lightly with your fingertips.

Bake for 25 minutes until the edges begin to brown. Cool on a wire rack. Cut into 12 bars.

Makes 12 bars

High Fiber, Low Heart Attacks

Research on nearly twenty-two thousand male smokers in Finland found that those with the highest fiber intake (averaging about 35 grams a day) suffered one third fewer heart attacks over a six-year period. Furthermore, for every 10 gram increase in dietary fiber, the risk from coronary death fell by 17 percent.
Circulation 94(11):2720–2727, 1996

Stir-fried Rice

The brown rice and bulgur mixture can be made a day ahead. Once you start stir-frying, the recipe goes very fast.

THE SNEAK:

- Fried rice is usually a brownish color because of the soy sauce. This dish is brown, however, because of its whole grains. The bulgur especially helps to kick up the fiber content.

NUTRITION SCORECARD (PER SERVING)		NOTABLE NUTRIENT (PER SERVING)	AMOUNT	% DAILY VALUE
Calories	112			
Fat (grams)	1.4			
% Fat calories	10			
Protein (grams)	4	Fiber (grams)	4	16
Carbohydrates (grams)	23			
Cholesterol (milligrams)	0			

- ½ cup instant brown rice
- ½ cup bulgur (cracked wheat)
- 1 cup chicken broth
- 2 egg whites
- 1 whole egg
- ½ teaspoon mustard powder
- 2 cloves garlic
- 1 teaspoon shredded fresh ginger
- 1 cup shredded cabbage
- ⅓ cup shredded carrot
- ¼ cup chopped chives
- 1 (8-ounce) can sliced water chestnuts, drained
- 2 tablespoons reduced sodium soy sauce
- 1 teaspoon dark sesame oil

In a medium saucepan combine the brown rice, bulgur, and chicken broth. Bring to a boil and reduce the heat. Cover and simmer for 15 minutes until the liquid is absorbed. Remove from the heat. Cool to room temperature, or cover and refrigerate until ready to use.

In a small bowl beat together the egg whites, whole egg, and dry mustard until blended. Lightly coat a large skillet or wok with nonstick vegetable spray. Over medium heat add the beaten eggs. Cook the eggs without stirring until they begin to set; stir and cook until the egg bits are small and crumbly. Remove and set aside.

Slightly cook the skillet, then spray it again with nonstick spray. Add the garlic and ginger. Cook and stir over medium-high heat until fragrant, about 1 minute. Add the cabbage, carrot, and chives. Cook and stir for about 3 minutes until the vegetables are tender. Stir in the cooked rice mixture, scrambled egg bits, and water chestnuts. Cook and stir until heated through, about 3 minutes. Combine the soy sauce and sesame oil and add to the rice mixture. Cook and stir for 2 minutes.

Makes 6 side-dish servings

Chicken Bundles with Apricot Stuffing and Honey-Orange Sauce

You'll want to serve this meal for company—it's so good. The stuffing is studded with dried apricots and simmered in orange juice.

THE SNEAK:

- Bulgur (cracked wheat) is the basis for the stuffing.

NUTRITION SCORECARD (PER SERVING)		NOTABLE NUTRIENT (PER SERVING)	AMOUNT	% DAILY VALUE
Calories	319			
Fat (grams)	3.5			
% Fat calories	10			
Protein (grams)	30	Fiber (grams)	5	20
Carbohydrates (grams)	43			
Cholesterol (milligrams)	73			

Apricot Stuffing

- ½ cup bulgur (cracked wheat)
- 1 cup orange juice
- 2 tablespoons minced onion
- 2 tablespoons chopped celery
- 2 tablespoons diced dried apricot
- ½ teaspoon dried sage
- ½ teaspoon dried marjoram
- 2 tablespoons chopped parsley

Chicken

- 4 boneless, skinless chicken breasts

Honey-Orange Sauce

- ¼ cup honey
- ¼ cup orange juice
- 3 tablespoons reduced-sodium soy sauce
- 1 teaspoon cornstarch
- 4 (¼-inch) orange slices

To Make the Stuffing: In a small saucepan combine the bulgur, orange juice, onion, celery, apricot, sage, and marjoram. Bring to a boil and reduce the heat. Cover and simmer for 15 minutes until the liquid is absorbed. Remove from the heat. Stir in the parsley.

Meanwhile, prepare the chicken breasts. Rinse the chicken and pat dry. Place each breast between 2 pieces of clear plastic wrap. Working from the center to the edges, lightly pound the chicken with the flat side of a meat mallet to form ⅛-inch-thick rectangles.

Preheat the oven to 350°F.

Place ¼ of the stuffing on each chicken piece. Fold in the long sides of the chicken and roll up jelly-roll style, beginning at one of the short sides. Secure with wooden toothpicks. Place the chicken bundles in a 10-inch square baking dish. Bake 30 to 35 minutes until the chicken is no longer pink.

To make the Honey-Orange Sauce: In a small saucepan stir together the honey, orange juice, and 2 tablespoons soy sauce. Cook over medium heat. Stir together the remaining 1 tablespoon soy sauce with cornstarch until smooth. Add to the honey mixture. Cook and stir until the mixture is thickened and bubbly.

Transfer the chicken bundles to a serving plate. Pour the sauce over the bundles. Garnish with orange slices and serve.

Makes 4 servings

Streusel Coffee Cake

One bite of this and you'll be sure to lick the crumbs off the plate. I wish I could say that I was clever enough to come up with this sneak, but I was inspired when I came across this flourless barley coffee cake recipe by syndicated columnist Cathy Thomas of the Orange County Register. *I adapted it to be lower in fat and calories. By the way, this can be made totally wheat-free by just omitting the wheat germ—quality will not suffer. Note: Be sure to plan ahead for this recipe because the barley needs to be soaked overnight.*

THE SNEAK:

- Barley! Barley is soaked and ground in a food processor. Wheat germ is added to the streusel to add a bit more fiber. Oats are added as a decorative topping as well as to contribute fiber.

NUTRITION SCORECARD (PER SERVING)		NOTABLE NUTRIENT (PER SERVING)	AMOUNT	% DAILY VALUE
Calories	200	Fiber (grams)	4	16
Fat (grams)	4.1			
% Fat calories	18			
Protein (grams)	5			
Carbohydrates (grams)	37			
Cholesterol (milligrams)	3			

1 cup pearl barley
1 1/3 cups water

STREUSEL

1/2 cup brown sugar
3 tablespoons wheat germ
1 1/2 teaspoons cinnamon
2 tablespoons light butter, melted

CAKE

3/4 cup brown sugar
3 tablespoons fat-free sour cream
1 teaspoon baking powder
1/2 teaspoon ground cinnamon
1/4 teaspoon nutmeg
1/4 teaspoon salt
3 egg whites

TOPPING

2 tablespoons oats
1/3 cup chopped pecans

Soak the barley in water overnight for at least 8 hours. Spray a 9-inch springform pan with nonstick vegetable spray.

To make the streusel: In a small bowl mix together the brown sugar, wheat germ, and cinnamon. Stir in the melted light butter. Set aside.

To make the cake: Place the barley and soaking water in a food processor fitted with the metal blade. Process until finely and uniformly ground, resembling cooked oatmeal. Add the 3/4 cup brown sugar, sour cream, baking powder, cinnamon, nutmeg, and salt.

In a large bowl beat the egg whites with an electric mixer on high setting until soft peaks form, about 2 minutes. Add the barley mixture and beat until blended. Note: The batter will appear runny.

To assemble: Preheat the oven to 350°F. Spoon half the batter into the prepared pan. Using your fingertips, sprinkle half of the streusel mixture over the batter. Drop the remaining batter by spoonfuls over the streusel layer, and carefully spread the batter evenly, using the back of a spoon. Using your fingertips, sprinkle the remaining streusel over the batter. Sprinkle the oats and pecans evenly over the top. Bake for 30 to 35 minutes. Remove from the oven and cool. To serve, run a knife around the sides of the pan to loosen the cake. Release the pan sides. Cut into 9 pieces.

Makes 9 servings

Low-Fiber Diet May Lead to Diabetes

A study examining the eating habits of more than sixty-five thousand women aged forty to sixty-five found that women who ate the lowest amount of fiber had two and a half times as great a risk of developing diabetes.
Journal of the American Medical Association 277(6):427–477, 1997

✖ Cinnayum Rolls ✖

When these goodies are baking in the oven, their heavenly cinnamon scent will beckon long lost friends from miles around. The sour cream in the dough also adds a wonderful flavor. This is a delicious treat or breakfast delight.

THE SNEAK:

- Whole wheat flour is incorporated and camouflaged with specks of spice in the dough and a ribbon of cinnamon and brown sugar, and crowned with a powdered sugar glaze.

NUTRITION SCORECARD (PER SERVING—1 ROLL)		NOTABLE NUTRIENT (PER SERVING—1 ROLL)		
Calories	217			
Fat (grams)	2.3		AMOUNT	% DAILY VALUE
% Fat calories	9			
Protein (grams)	7	Fiber (grams)	3.5	14
Carbohydrates (grams)	43			
Cholesterol (milligrams)	24			

DOUGH

1	cup fat-free sour cream
3	tablespoons white sugar
1	package active dry yeast
1/2	teaspoon salt
1/8	teaspoon baking soda
1	egg
1 1/2	cups whole wheat flour
1 1/2	cups all-purpose flour
1/2	teaspoon ground cinnamon
1/2	teaspoon ground nutmeg
1/4	teaspoon ground cloves

FILLING

1/3	cup brown sugar
1 1/2	teaspoons ground cinnamon
2	tablespoons light butter, melted

GLAZE

1/4	cup powdered sugar
1/4	teaspoon vanilla
1	to 1 1/2 teaspoons nonfat milk

To make the dough: In a small saucepan cook the sour cream over medium-low heat, stirring constantly just until the sour cream is warm. (Do not boil and do not try heating in the microwave or the sour cream will curdle.) Remove from the heat.

Transfer the heated sour cream to a large mixing bowl. Stir in the white sugar, yeast, salt, and baking soda until dissolved. Using a wooden spoon, stir in the egg.

Combine the whole wheat flour, all-purpose flour, ½ teaspoon ground cinnamon, nutmeg, and cloves. Add as much of this flour mixture to the sour cream mixture as you can.

Turn the dough out onto a floured surface and knead the dough for 6 to 8 minutes, incorporating enough of the remaining flour as needed to produce a dough that is smooth and elastic. Shape the dough into a ball; cover and let rest for 10 minutes.

In a small bowl, combine the brown sugar and cinnamon. Set aside.

Lightly spray a baking sheet with nonstick vegetable spray and set aside.

On a lightly floured surface roll out the dough to a 20- × 10-inch rectangle. Brush the dough with the melted light butter. Sprinkle the brown sugar mixture evenly over the dough.

Starting at the short side, roll up the dough to form a cylinder (the length will be 10 inches long). Pinch the seam together to seal. With the seam side down, cut each roll into 10 equal pieces and transfer to the prepared baking sheet. Cover and let rise until almost double in size (about 1 hour). Meanwhile, preheat the oven to 375°.

Uncover the rolls and bake for 12 to 15 minutes until lightly browned. Cool slightly and transfer to a serving platter.

To make the glaze: In a small bowl, stir together the powdered sugar, vanilla, and enough milk to make a glaze of the desired consistency. Drizzle the glaze over the warm rolls and serve.

Makes 10 rolls

Try These Other Fiber-Rich Recipes

CHAPTER SEVEN

Iron Men and Maidens

Why Iron Is Hot

Iron deficiency is the most common form of malnutrition in the world, affecting about 2.15 billion people. In the United States, iron deficiency is still very common. In fact, a disturbing report shows how widespread the problem is, affecting:

- 7.8 million adolescent girls and women of childbearing years
- nearly 1 million toddlers

Iron is such a concern that it is one of three key nutrients targeted for improvement by the Healthy People 2000 (the national prevention initiative to improve the health of all Americans by the year 2000).

ROLE OF IRON—BEYOND IRON-POOR BLOOD

Energy. You may already be familiar with one role that iron plays—energy. Iron helps to carry oxygen to the blood and deliver it to hungry cells. When you don't have enough iron, the red blood cells can't carry as much oxygen, and you'll wind up feeling sluggish and tired. Even marginal iron deficiency, which is not yet severe enough to be anemia, can affect physical performance.

Cold Streak. Iron is the key nutrient that regulates the body's ability to produce heat. So if you feel cold all the time, no matter how many layers of clothes you wear, inadequate iron could be the culprit.

Mind Games—Learning, Memory, and Behavior. Iron plays a critical role in the brain. The brain has the highest metabolic rate of any organ and requires high levels of iron and oxygen. Iron is essential to brain growth and development. It also regulates many brain hormones, including the neurotransmitters serotonin and dopamine. It should be no surprise that compelling studies on children show that iron deficiency can affect learning, memory, and behavior that could persist throughout life. There are studies under way to see if this is reversible and if it occurs at other stages of life.

MAKING THE MOST OUT OF THE IRON IN YOUR FOOD: IRON ENHANCERS

Enhancing iron absorption is like trying to earn maximum interest on an investment or savings account. If you eat iron under the right conditions, your body will actually retain more of it. The two key iron enhancers are vitamin C and meat.

Vitamin C. Eating vitamin C-rich foods at a meal can dramatically boost iron absorption by two- to four-fold. This is especially helpful for vegetarians.

Meats, Seafood, and Poultry. These contain a super-special type of iron called heme iron, which is highly absorbable—up to fifteen times higher than any other form of iron in the diet. The other type of iron in the diet (and the most prevalent) is called nonheme iron and only 2 to 20 percent of it is absorbed. Not only does meat contain this special type of iron but it also offers another advantage: Its protein enhances iron absorption. It has been estimated that every gram of meat eaten with a meal enhances iron absorption equivalent to 1 milligram of vitamin C. So let's say you add a little beef to a vegetable stirfry. The presence of beef will increase the amount of iron that gets from the vegetables into your bloodstream.

Iron Cookware—Grandma's Pans. I'll never forget learning about the Bantu Indians; they were famous for brewing beer in huge iron kettles. It is from this tribe that we learned that iron gets leached from pots into our food. I am not suggesting that you set up a little home brewery to enrich your diet with iron. But if you cook with an iron skillet you can add a considerable amount of iron to your meals. For example, spaghetti sauce that is simmered in an iron pan has *twenty-nine times* the iron content as the same spaghetti sauce cooked in glassware.

IRONING OUT THE DETAILS—HOW MUCH IRON?

Iron demands are at their greatest during periods of rapid growth such as childhood and adolescence, and childbearing years for women and pregnancy. You really get an appreciation for this demand when you look at a toddler's iron needs. Children aged one through ten have the *identical* iron requirement as a grown man, 10 milligrams per day. Here's what you need according to age and gender, based on the Recommended Dietary Allowances:

AGE	GENDER	IRON (milligrams)
1–10	Boys and girls	10
11–18	Male	12
19 and older	Male	10
11–50	Female	15
51 and older	Female	10
Pregnant	Female (obviously)	30

GETTING MORE IRON IN YOUR DIET

Don't be afraid to add a little red meat to your cooking. Ironically, since many women have shunned red meat in the interest of low-fat eating, iron intakes have declined. It's still possible to eat a low-fat diet with red meat. Keep in mind with poultry, that the dark meat is higher in iron. The darker the meat, the higher the iron. This is because the deep red color comes from hemoglobin. And the more hemoglobin, the higher the precious heme iron content.

Five Ways to Sneak Iron into Meals

1. Beef it up a bit—top round steak is the leanest cut of beef and a good source of iron. Try the Fiesta Fajitas, page 179.

2. Oysters and clams—now you have another reason to indulge in seafood. Oysters and clams in particular are loaded in iron. Try the Manhattan (Red) Clam Chowder, page 176.

3. Explore the dark side—don't be afraid to opt for dark meat poultry occasionally. The French Toast Turkey-Ham Sandwiches on page 177 take advantage of turkey ham, which comes from the dark meat or thigh.

4. Vegetarian options—you don't have to have meat to get a good iron source. Try the delicious Spiced Gingerbread on page 190.

5. Include a high vitamin C food—the Chili-Stuffed Potatoes, page 189, is a good example. The potato is a good source of vitamin C, which enhances the iron absorption from the chili.

Iron-Rich Foods

Food	Iron (milligrams)
Baked potato, 1	2.8
Beef pot roast, 4 ounces cooked	4.3
Cashews, ¼ cup	2.1
Clams, ¼ cup canned, drained	11.2
Cocoa powder, ¼ cup	3.0
Dried beans, 1 cup cooked	2.5–6.6
Green peas, 1 cup cooked	2.5
Jerusalem artichoke, 1 cup raw	5.1
Molasses, dark ½ cup	7.8
Oysters, ¼ cup canned	4.2
Peach halves, 10 each dried	5.3
Pistachio nuts, ¼ cup	2.2
Prune juice, 1 cup	3.0
Sesame seeds, 2 tablespoons	2.6
Snow pea pods, 1 cup raw	3.0
Tomato paste, ½ cup	3.9
Top round steak, 4 ounces cooked	3.2
Turkey, dark meat, 4 ounces	2.7

Source: Computer nutrition analysis using Food Processor v2.2 software

---

Stainless Steel, Too, Contributes Iron

Cooking in stainless steel pans can significantly increase the iron content of food. Stainless steel is an alloy metal that contains 50 to 80 percent iron. The longer the cooking time and the more acidic the food (such as tomato sauce), the more iron will be leached from the pan and into the food. Stainless steel cookware accounts for 43 percent of all cookware sold.
Journal of the American Dietetic Association 97(6):659–661, 1997

Twenty Ways to Increase Iron in Your Diet

1. Add dried fruits to your favorite cereals.
2. Eat or drink a vitamin C-rich food with your meals to increase iron absorption.
3. Try a snack of smoked oysters (heme iron) and whole grain crackers.
4. Order a bowl of red clam chowder (heme iron) at your favorite restaurant. The red or Manhattan variety is much lower in fat.
5. Add lean beef (heme iron) to a spaghetti sauce.
6. In the mood for a burger? Go for the smallest and you'll raise your iron while keeping your fat intake low.
7. Cook in an iron skillet.
8. Try dark molasses as a moist sweetener instead of honey.
9. Add chopped bell peppers to chili—the extra vitamin C will increase iron absorption.
10. Have a wedge of cantaloupe (high C food) with iron-fortified breakfast cereal.
11. Don't drink coffee or tea in between meals. These beverages interfere with iron absorption.
12. Have a sweet tooth? Try *real* black licorice—one serving provides 15 percent of the Daily Value for iron!
13. Add green bell pepper (high C) slices to a lean roast beef sandwich.
14. Top a spinach salad with mandarin oranges (high C).
15. Add a generous helping of fresh salsa (high C) to a bean burrito.
16. Keep a stash of dried peach halves for a convenient snack.
17. Throw some toasted sesame seeds on a Chinese chicken salad. The heme iron from the chicken and the vitamin C from the greens will increase the iron absorption from the sesame seeds.
18. If you are taking an iron supplement, do not drink milk with it or take a calcium supplement. Calcium interferes with iron absorption.
19. Try fish for a lean entree—it has both heme iron and a type of protein that enhances iron absorption.
20. Serve a fresh fruit tart with kiwi and strawberries for dessert. Not only is it a pleasant way to finish off a meal but its high vitamin C will boost iron absorption.

Accidental Iron Overdose and Kids

Accidental iron overdose is the leading cause of poisoning deaths in children under age six. Since 1986, the poison control centers in the United States have received reports of more than 110,000 incidents of children under six accidentally swallowing iron tablets. Some of the children were hospitalized and more than thirty-five died. The children were poisoned after consuming as few as five to as many as ninety-eight iron-containing pills. Death occurred from ingesting as little as 200 milligrams to nearly 6,000 milligrams of iron. To put these levels into perspective, the Recommended Dietary Allowance for children six months to ten years is 10 milligrams.

Iron supplements (or iron-containing supplements) are normally safe when taken at the proper dose. They are particularly valuable when this essential mineral is lacking in the diet, a common problem especially for women of childbearing years and children.

Iron poisoning symptoms include both immediate and long-term problems:

• Immediate symptoms can include nausea, vomiting, diarrhea, and gastrointestinal bleeding which can progress to shock, coma, and death.

• Long-term symptoms can occur three to six weeks after the poisoning even if the child appears to have recovered. These include liver damage and gastrointestinal obstruction.

The FDA recommends two key steps to prevent accidental iron overdose:

• Always keep iron-containing products out of reach of children.

• Completely re-close child-resistant packages of iron-containing products every time they are opened.

If a child has accidentally swallowed a product that contains iron, parents should contact a doctor or local poison control center immediately, even if there are no immediate symptoms. Sometimes, serious symptoms do not develop right away.

�֎ Manhattan (Red) Clam Chowder �֎

It is rare for one meal, let alone one dish, to provide more than 100 percent of your iron needs—but this one does! Clams are naturally high in iron so this recipe was tweaked only to modify fat.

THE SNEAK:

• Using a familiar recipe with naturally iron-rich clams

NUTRITION SCORECARD (PER SERVING)		NOTABLE NUTRIENT (PER SERVING)		
Calories	176			
Fat (grams)	1.6		AMOUNT	% DAILY VALUE
% Fat calories	8			
Protein (grams)	15	Iron (milligrams)	19.4	108
Carbohydrates (grams)	20			
Cholesterol (milligrams)	44			

2	cups fat-free chicken broth	⅛	teaspoon black pepper
2	cups diced potatoes	4	(6½-ounce) cans minced clams (with juices)
½	cup diced carrots		
½	cup diced celery	1½	cups chopped fresh tomatoes or canned diced tomatoes
½	cup diced onion		
1	clove garlic, minced	1	(8-ounce) can tomato sauce
½	teaspoon dried thyme	¼	cup snipped parsley, loosely packed
¼	teaspoon dried oregano		

In a large saucepan combine the chicken broth, potatoes, carrots, celery, onion, garlic, thyme, oregano, and pepper. Bring to a boil. Reduce the heat and cover and cook about 20 minutes until the vegetables are tender.

Stir in the undrained clams, tomatoes, and tomato sauce. Heat until bubbly. Stir in the parsley and serve.

Makes 6 servings (1 ½ cups each)

✳ French Toast Turkey-Ham Sandwiches ✳

These breakfast sandwiches make a good meal any time of the day. They look particularly elegant when trimmed of their crusts (before being dipped into the egg bath) and cut into triangles after cooking.

THE SNEAK:

- The dark meat of the turkey, of which turkey ham is made (usually made of thigh meat), is a good source of iron.
- Serve this with a glass of orange juice and you will easily double the iron absorption.

NUTRITION SCORECARD (PER SERVING)		NOTABLE NUTRIENT (PER SERVING)		
			AMOUNT	% DAILY VALUE
Calories	361			
Fat (grams)	9.9			
% Fat calories	25			
Protein (grams)	35	Iron (milligrams)	4.9	27
Carbohydrates		Fiber (grams)	4	16
(grams)	34	Calcium (milligrams)	348	35
Cholesterol				
(milligrams)	111			

8	slices whole wheat bread, crusts trimmed if desired	1	large egg
12	slices (12 ounces) turkey ham	2	egg whites
4	slices (4 ounces) reduced-fat Swiss cheese (such as Alpine Lace or Jarlsberg)	2	tablespoons nonfat milk
			pinch of nutmeg

For each sandwich, layer 1 slice of bread with 1 slice of turkey ham, ½ slice of Swiss cheese, 1 slice of turkey ham, ½ slice of Swiss cheese, and 1 slice of turkey ham. Top with 1 slice of bread.

In a shallow dish beat the whole egg, egg whites, milk, and nutmeg.

Lightly coat a large griddle or skillet with nonstick spray and heat over medium heat.

Dip the sandwiches into the egg mixture to coat well on both sides. Cook the sandwiches in batches, if necessary, over medium heat for 3 to

4 minutes on each side, turning and pressing lightly with a spatula until golden brown.

Remove the sandwiches to serving plates. Cut in half or quarters and serve immediately.

Makes 4 sandwiches

What About Heart Disease and Men?

A 1992 study of two thousand middle-aged men in eastern Finland caused a big stir because it found that men with the most iron in their systems were more than twice as likely to suffer heart attacks compared to men with relatively low iron reserves. Most studies since, however, have been unable to confirm this connection. The latest research not only discounts the Finnish study but poses the possibility that low iron levels may increase the risk of heart disease. Researchers at the National Institute of Aging found that men with the *most* iron in their blood had a significantly lower risk of dying from heart disease; in fact, they had one fifth the risk compared to men with the lowest concentrations of iron.

Tufts University Health & Nutrition Letter 15(3):3, 1997

❈ Fiesta Fajitas ❈

This simple meal is easy to make and sure to please. Tip: It's much easier to slice the meat into thin strips if it is partially frozen.

THE SNEAK:

- Lean beef is used for its high iron content in a highly absorbable form. The vitamin C-rich peppers also increase iron absorption.

NUTRITION SCORECARD (PER SERVING)		NOTABLE NUTRIENT (PER SERVING)		
Calories	432			
Fat (grams)	6		AMOUNT	% DAILY VALUE
% Fat calories	12			
Protein (grams)	37	Iron (milligrams)	5.3	29
Carbohydrates		Vitamin C (milligrams)	134	223
(grams)	60	Fiber (grams)	8	32
Cholesterol				
(milligrams)	71			

¼	teaspoon ground cumin	1	clove garlic, minced
¼	teaspoon chili powder	¼	cup snipped fresh cilantro
¼	teaspoon dried oregano	1	tablespoon lime juice
¼	teaspoon salt	1	pound top round steak, cut into thin strips
1	medium onion, sliced	¼	teaspoon crushed red pepper flakes
1	medium green bell pepper, seeded and cut into long, thin strips	12	small flour tortillas (7-inch diameter)
1	medium red bell pepper, seeded and cut into long, thin strips		
1	medium yellow bell pepper, seeded and cut into long, thin strips		

In a small bowl stir together the cumin, chili powder, oregano, and salt. Set aside.

Spray a large skillet or wok with nonstick cooking spray. Add the onion, green bell pepper, red bell pepper, yellow bell pepper, and garlic. Cook and stir over medium heat just until the vegetables are tender. Add the cilantro, lime juice, and cumin spice mixture. Cook and stir for 2 minutes. Using a slotted spoon, transfer the vegetable mixture to a large bowl and set aside.

Increase the heat to medium-high. Add the steak and red pepper flakes. Cook and stir until the beef reaches the desired doneness, about 5 minutes.

Return the vegetables to the skillet and heat through. Serve with the tortillas.

Makes 4 servings (3 fajitas each)

✕ Spaghetti with Sun-Dried Tomato Sauce ✕

If you like a little kick to your spaghetti sauce be sure to use the "hot" turkey sausage. Like many spaghetti sauces, the longer it cooks the better it tastes (just be sure to keep the lid on the pan while the sauce is simmering).

THE SNEAK:

• There are many iron contributors to this meal: sun-dried tomatoes, tomato paste, turkey sausage, and the pasta. Together they add up to a significant source of iron.

NUTRITION SCORECARD (PER SERVING)		NOTABLE NUTRIENT (PER SERVING)		
Calories	365			
Fat (grams)	7.0		AMOUNT	% DAILY VALUE
% Fat calories	17			
Protein (grams)	18	Iron (milligrams)	4.9	27
Carbohydrates (grams)	60			
Cholesterol (milligrams)	29			

2	(3-ounce) links lean turkey sausage (hot or sweet), casing removed	1	(6-ounce) can tomato paste
		1	teaspoon dried basil
½	cup chopped onion	½	teaspoon dried oregano
1	green bell pepper, chopped	1	teaspoon dried thyme
3	cloves garlic, minced	1	teaspoon sugar
1	(28-ounce) can diced tomatoes, undrained	12	ounces spaghetti noodles
		6	tablespoons freshly grated Parmesan cheese
½	cup sun-dried tomatoes, diced		

Spray a 4-quart pan with nonstick vegetable spray. Add the turkey sausage, onion, bell pepper, and garlic. Cook and stir until the turkey is cooked through and no longer pink. Stir in the undrained canned tomatoes, sun-dried tomatoes, tomato paste, basil, oregano, thyme, and sugar. Bring to a boil. Reduce the heat. Cover and simmer for at least 30 minutes.

Meanwhile, just before you are ready to serve, cook the spaghetti noodles according to the manufacturer's directions and drain well. Transfer the noodles to a serving platter, top with spaghetti sauce and Parmesan, and serve.

Makes 6 servings

Physical Fitness Is Tough Without Enough Iron

Healthy active women with iron deficiency, but not severe enough to be anemia, showed significantly diminished physical performance compared to women with adequate iron stores.
American Journal of Clinical Nutrition 66(2):334–341, 1997

Cold Capellini with Cajun Clam Sauce

This feisty sauce will liven up your taste buds. This is best made the night before to allow the flavors to meld.

THE SNEAK:

- Clams are a great source of iron. The strong flavors from the garlic, parsley, and peppers will alleviate any worries of a "fishy" taste.

NUTRITION SCORECARD (PER SERVING)		NOTABLE NUTRIENT (PER SERVING)		
Calories	428			
Fat (grams)	4.3		AMOUNT	% DAILY VALUE
% Fat calories	9			
Protein (grams)	36	Iron (milligrams)	30.2	168
Carbohydrates (grams)	57			
Cholesterol (milligrams)	67			

- 1 teaspoon olive oil
- 2/3 cup chopped parsley
- 10 cloves garlic, minced
- 4 (6½-ounce) cans chopped clams, drained (reserve juices)
- ½ cup evaporated skim milk, divided
- ¼ cup dry white wine
- 1 tablespoon white Worcestershire sauce
- ½ teaspoon salt
- ¼ teaspoon white pepper
- ¼ teaspoon red cayenne pepper
- 8 ounces angel hair pasta
- 4 teaspoons cornstarch

Spray a 4-quart pan with nonstick olive oil spray. Add the olive oil. Add the chopped parsley and garlic. Cook and stir over medium-high heat until fragrant, about 1 minute. Add the reserved clam juices, ¼ cup evaporated milk, wine, Worcestershire, salt, white pepper, and cayenne pepper. Bring to a boil. Reduce the heat and simmer for 10 minutes, uncovered.

Meanwhile, cook the pasta according to the manufacturer's directions and drain.

Mix together the cornstarch and the remaining evaporated milk until smooth. Add to the sauce. Cook and stir until thickened, about 1 minute.

Add the chopped clams and the cooked pasta to the sauce. Cook and stir until heated through. Transfer to a large serving bowl. Cover and chill overnight.

Makes 4 servings

Iron Affects Memory and Learning

A study looking at the effects of iron deficiency without anemia in adolescent girls found that those who received an iron supplement during an eight-week period performed significantly better on a test of verbal learning and memory than iron-deficient girls who received a placebo pill. Iron deficiency without anemia is a very early stage of malnutrition in which the red blood cells are not yet affected by an inadequate iron intake.

Lancet 348:992–996, 1996

One-Pot Chili Mac

This one-dish meal is easy to put together and tastes great left over (if there are any leftovers).

THE SNEAK:

- Lean meat (ground turkey or extra lean beef) combined with kidney beans makes this a fiber-rich as well as iron-rich meal.

NUTRITION SCORECARD (PER SERVING)	WITH GROUND TURKEY	WITH EXTRA LEAN GROUND BEEF	NOTABLE NUTRIENT (PER SERVING)	AMOUNT	% DAILY VALUE
Calories	376	398	Fiber (grams)	12	48
Fat (grams)	10.4	12	Iron (milligrams)		
% Fat calories	258	27	w/ground turkey	4.9	27

NUTRITION SCORECARD (PER SERVING)			NOTABLE NUTRIENT (PER SERVING)		
	WITH GROUND TURKEY	WITH EXTRA LEAN GROUND BEEF		AMOUNT	% DAILY VALUE
Protein (grams)	28	28	Iron (milligrams)		
Carbohydrates (grams)	44	44	w/ground extra lean beef	5.3	30
Cholesterol (milligrams)	65	67			

1 pound ground turkey or extra lean ground beef
1 cup chopped onions
2 cloves garlic, minced
2 teaspoons chili powder
1 teaspoon ground cumin
1 (28-ounce) can red kidney beans, drained

2 (8-ounce) cans tomato sauce
1 (14½-ounce) can diced tomatoes, with juices
¼ cup tomato paste
¾ cup small elbow macaroni
¼ cup water
½ cup finely shredded reduced-fat sharp Cheddar cheese

Spray a 4-quart pan with nonstick vegetable spray. Add the ground meat, onions, garlic, chili, and cumin. Cook and stir occasionally until the meat is cooked through and no longer pink.

Stir in the drained beans, tomato sauce, tomatoes, and tomato paste. Add the macaroni and water. Bring to a boil, then reduce the heat. Cover and simmer for 10 minutes. Stir well, then cover and simmer for about 10 minutes more until the macaroni is tender but firm. Stir occasionally. Remove the lid and sprinkle with the cheese. Cover and heat over low heat until the cheese melts. Serve.

Makes 6 hearty servings

✖ Beef Stroganoff ✖

This scrumptious stroganoff gets a head start by using a low-fat cream of mushroom soup. While I have been disappointed in many fat-free and low-fat products, the cream soups are surprisingly good.

THE SNEAK:

- Lean beef is used for its high heme iron content (a highly absorbable form of iron).

NUTRITION SCORECARD (PER SERVING)		NOTABLE NUTRIENT (PER SERVING)		
Calories	471			
Fat (grams)	7.3		AMOUNT	% DAILY VALUE
% Fat calories	14			
Protein (grams)	40	Iron (milligrams)	4.8	27
Carbohydrates (grams)	59			
Cholesterol (milligrams)	78			

4 cups (8 ounces) dry bow-ties or yolk-free egg noodles
1 pound top round steak, *trimmed of all visible fat*
1 teaspoon Hungarian paprika
½ cup chopped onion
2 cloves garlic, minced

2 cups sliced mushrooms
1 (10¾ ounces) can condensed reduced-fat cream of mushroom soup
¼ teaspoon black pepper
¾ cup fat-free sour cream

Cook the noodles according to the manufacturer's directions. Cut the steak across the grain into thin bite-size pieces and sprinkle with paprika. Meanwhile, spray a skillet with nonstick vegetable spray. Add the beef, onion, and garlic. Cook and stir for 3 minutes. Add the mushrooms. Cook and stir until the beef is no longer pink and the mushrooms are tender. Reduce the heat to low.

Stir in the soup and pepper. Cover and simmer for 5 minutes. Remove the skillet from the heat. Stir in the sour cream and serve right away over the cooked noodles.

Makes 4 servings

Restless Leg Syndrome (RLS)

RLS is characterized by an irresistible urge to move the legs, which are relieved by movement. While RLS affects only 5 to 8 percent of Americans, a whopping 30 percent of individuals with iron deficiency is affected. The severity of symptoms from this disorder correlates to an iron status biomarker, ferritin. The lower the ferritin the more severe the symptoms.

Nutrition Today 32(3):102–109, 1997

Chinese Beef Broccoli with Snow Peas

This is a quick and easy meal to make. Once again, to make the task of cutting thin slices of beef easier, it helps to partially freeze the meat first. The beef strips can be marinated overnight; just be sure to cover and refrigerate until you are ready to cook.

THE SNEAK:

- Lean beef is used for its high iron content in a highly absorbable form. The vitamin C-rich broccoli and snow peas also increase iron absorption.

NUTRITION SCORECARD (PER SERVING)		NOTABLE NUTRIENT (PER SERVING)	AMOUNT	% DAILY VALUE
Calories	437			
Fat (grams)	9.5			
% Fat calories	20			
Protein (grams)	38	Iron (milligrams)	5.7	32
Carbohydrates (grams)	50	Fiber (grams)	7	28
Cholesterol (milligrams)	71			

1 pound top round steak, slightly frozen
1 teaspoon grated ginger
1 pound broccoli florets
½ pound snow pea pods

MARINADE
  2   tablespoons oyster sauce
  1   tablespoon dry sherry
  1   tablespoon light soy sauce
  1   teaspoon cornstarch
  1   tablespoon sesame oil
  1   teaspoon sugar
  1   clove garlic, minced

SAUCE
  2   teaspoons cornstarch
  2/3 cup beef broth
  1   tablespoon light soy sauce
  1/4 teaspoon pepper
  3   cups cooked brown rice

Slice the beef across the grain and at an angle into thin strips. In a shallow dish mix together the oyster sauce, dry sherry, 1 tablespoon light soy sauce, 1 teaspoon cornstarch, sesame oil, and sugar. Add the beef strips and mix well to coat. Let stand for 30 minutes.

Spray a wok or large skillet with nonstick vegetable spray. Stir-fry marinated beef until no longer pink, about 3 minutes. With a slotted spoon remove the cooked beef (the juices will remain).

Add the garlic and ginger to the wok. Cook and stir until fragrant, about 30 seconds. Add the broccoli. Cook and stir for 3 minutes. Add the snow peas and cook for 2 minutes.

In a small bowl combine the 2 teaspoons cornstarch, broth, 1 tablespoon light soy sauce, and pepper. Mix thoroughly until smooth. Add the cornstarch mixture to the broccoli mixture. Cook and stir until the sauce thickens slightly, about 2 minutes. Add the cooked beef and mix well until heated through. Remove and serve with rice.

Makes 4 servings

Ferritin—The Gold Standard of Blood Iron Tests

One of the most reliable and sensitive tests to assess your iron status is ferritin. Unfortunately, it is not routinely drawn with standard blood work. Ferritin is the storage form of iron. Therefore even if the levels are low, it's not too late to increase your iron intake *before* getting anemia. It's much easier to prevent a deficiency than to correct it. If you wait to see changes in the conventional blood tests, usually hemoglobin, it's like waiting to get an "overdrawn" notice from your bank to add more funds to your account.
Annual Review of Nutrition 6:13–40, 1986

Old-fashioned Stuffing with Smoked Oysters

I prefer using crumbly stuffing mix rather than cubed because it melds nicely after cooking. But you can certainly use the cubed style if that's your preference. The dressing is finished with a little light butter which adds a nice rich flavor but not much fat.

THE SNEAK:

- Oysters are loaded with iron. Using a smoked variety adds a special flavor, while finely chopping them allows for a subtle presence with each bite.

NUTRITION SCORECARD (PER SERVING)	
Calories	245
Fat (grams)	3.8
% Fat calories	14
Protein (grams)	13
Carbohydrates (grams)	40
Cholesterol (milligrams)	30

NOTABLE NUTRIENT (PER SERVING)	AMOUNT	% DAILY VALUE
Iron (milligrams)	5.31	30
Vitamin A (RE)	255	26

- 1 cup chopped celery
- 1 cup sliced mushrooms
- ½ cup chopped onion
- 1 medium carrot, finely chopped or shredded
- 3 (3¾-ounce) cans smoked oysters, drained and chopped
- 1½ to 2 cups chicken broth
- 12 ounces seasoned stuffing mix
- 2 tablespoons melted light butter

Spray a 4-quart pan with nonstick vegetable spray. Add the celery, mushrooms, onion, and carrot. Cook and stir until tender. Stir in the chopped smoked oysters. Add 1½ cups chicken broth and bring to a boil. Remove the pan from the heat. Stir in the stuffing mix, tossing lightly. Cover and let stand for 5 minutes. Drizzle the melted light butter and toss lightly with a fork to fluff. If a moister dressing is desired, gradually drizzle in the remaining chicken broth.

Makes 8 hearty servings

✳ Chili-Stuffed Potatoes ✳

*I knew this recipe was a winner when my daughter asked
for seconds. The beauty of the dish is its ease of preparation.
When I'm in a hurry I'll speed things up a bit by first cooking the
potatoes in the microwave (5 to 7 minutes) and finishing them
in the oven for about 10 minutes.
You can use any low-fat canned chili and
beans, with options galore from turkey, chicken, beef, to vegetarian.
I used the vegetarian variety for those who are trying to boost
their iron intake without the use of meat. The chilis that
contain some type of animal protein do have
a higher iron content.*

THE SNEAK:

- The iron is incorporated by both the baked potato (with the skin) and the chili.

NUTRITION SCORECARD (PER SERVING)		NOTABLE NUTRIENT (PER SERVING)		
Calories	402			
Fat (grams)	3.6		AMOUNT	% DAILY VALUE
% Fat calories	8			
Protein (grams)	16	Iron (milligrams)	5.5	31
Carbohydrates		Fiber (grams)	14	56
(grams)	79			
Cholesterol				
(milligrams)	10			

4	medium potatoes (2 pounds)	4	tablespoons grated low-fat Cheddar cheese
2	cups canned low-fat vegetarian chili	1	medium tomato, diced
½	teaspoon Tabasco (optional)	¼	cup snipped chives

Scrub the potatoes well and pierce with a fork. Bake at 400°F for 45 to 50 minutes until fork tender.

Meanwhile, heat the chili according to the manufacturer's directions and add Tabasco if desired. Cut an X in each potato, then push the ends toward the center to open. Top each potato with ½ cup chili. Sprinkle the cheese, tomato, and chives on top and serve.

Makes 4 servings

✖ Spiced Gingerbread ✖

I no sooner made this treat than it was gone, lickety split, with neighbors and friends pleading for more, or at least the recipe. This rich and moist gingerbread gets its deep coloring from dark molasses, which happens to be a good source of iron.

THE SNEAK:

- Dark molasses for the iron
- As a little extra sneak, whole wheat flour is used for a fiber boost.
- Fat is cut by using a combination of buttermilk and applesauce.

NUTRITION SCORECARD (PER SLICE)		NOTABLE NUTRIENT (PER SERVING)		
Calories	258			
Fat (grams)	0.6		AMOUNT	% DAILY VALUE
% Fat calories	2			
Protein (grams)	5	Iron (milligrams)	6.9	38
Carbohydrates		Fiber (grams)	4	16
(grams)	63			
Cholesterol				
(milligrams)	1			

1¾	cups whole wheat flour	¼	teaspoon ground cloves
½	cup packed brown sugar	¼	teaspoon salt
2	teaspoons ginger	1	cup dark molasses
1	teaspoon cardamom	½	cup applesauce
½	teaspoon baking soda	⅓	cup buttermilk
¼	teaspoon cinnamon	2	egg whites

Preheat the oven to 350°F. Spray a 9-inch round cake pan with 2-inch high sides with nonstick vegetable spray.

In a large bowl combine the whole wheat flour, brown sugar, ginger, cardamom, baking soda, cinnamon, cloves, and salt.

In a medium bowl, using an electric mixer on slow speed, beat together the molasses, applesauce, buttermilk, and egg whites.

Add the molasses mixture to the flour mixture. Beat on medium speed until blended. Pour the batter into a prepared pan. Bake until the bread begins to pull away from the sides of the pan and a toothpick inserted into the center comes out clean, 40 to 45 minutes. Remove from the oven and cool on the rack for 10 minutes. Slice into 8 wedges. Tastes best served warm.

Makes 8 servings

Iron Deficiency Worsens Lead Poisoning

Several studies have shown that people who are iron deficient absorb more of the toxic mineral lead, making it easier to get lead poisoning.
American Journal of Clinical Nutrition 50(supplement):598–606, 1989

Harvest Granola with Dried Apricots and Cashews

This homemade granola beats any storebought version, and it's so easy to make. Eat as a snack, sprinkle over yogurt, or enjoy as a morning breakfast served with low-fat milk. Tip: Dip your scissors or knife into the oats before cutting the apricots—it prevents sticking.

THE SNEAK:

- The iron comes from a variety of sources: dried apricots, cashews, oats, and molasses—and such a delicious combination.

NUTRITION SCORECARD (PER SERVING)		NOTABLE NUTRIENT (PER SERVING)	AMOUNT	% DAILY VALUE
Calories	298			
Fat (grams)	10.2			
% Fat calories	29			
Protein (grams)	8	Iron (milligrams)	4.6	26
Carbohydrates (grams)	48	Fiber (grams)	5	20
Cholesterol (milligrams)	0			

- 2 1/2 cups regular rolled oats
- 3/4 cup cashew halves
- 1/2 cup wheat germ
- 1/3 cup sunflower seeds
- 1/3 cup dark molasses
- 1/3 cup honey
- 1 tablespoon canola oil
- 2 teaspoons cinnamon
- 1/2 teaspoon nutmeg
- 1 1/3 cups dried apricot halves, diced

Preheat the oven to 275°F. Spray a baking sheet or shallow pan with nonstick spray.

In a large bowl combine the oats, cashews, wheat germ, and sunflower seeds. In another small bowl stir together the molasses, honey, oil, cinnamon, and nutmeg. Drizzle over the oat mixture and toss well to coat. Spread the mixture evenly over the prepared pan.

Bake for 30 minutes until golden, stirring after 15 minutes and frequently thereafter to prevent burning. Remove from the oven and cool completely in the pan. Stir in the diced apricots. Store in an airtight container at room temperature for up to 2 weeks.

Makes 10 servings (about 5 cups, ¹/₂ cup each)

✖ Trail Mix with Chocolate Chip Bits ✖

The key to flavor in this satisfying snack lies in toasting the almonds and sesame seeds. Since this trail mix is made of tiny ingredients it's best eaten with a spoon. Try it over your favorite frozen yogurt— it tastes fantastic.

THE SNEAK:

• A combination of sources contributes to iron, including chocolate chips, almonds, dried fruits, and iron-fortified cereal.

NUTRITION SCORECARD (PER SERVING)		NOTABLE NUTRIENT (PER SERVING)		
Calories	268			
Fat (grams)	9.4		AMOUNT	% DAILY VALUE
% Fat calories	29			
Protein (grams)	7	Iron (milligrams)	5.8	32
Carbohydrates (grams)	45			
Cholesterol (milligrams)	0			

½	cup slivered almonds	1	cup Zante currants
3	tablespoons sesame seeds	½	cup mini chocolate chips
2	cups Grape Nuts or nugget-style cereal		

Preheat the oven to 350°F. Add the almonds and sesame seeds to a baking sheet. Bake, stirring occasionally, for about 5 minutes until golden and fragrant. Cool completely.

In a large bowl combine the cereal, currants, chocolate chips, and the cooled toasted almond mixture.

Makes 8 servings (1/2 cup each)

Coffee and Iron Don't Mix

Better not chase your iron supplement down with coffee. Coffee contains tannins which bind to iron in the intestine. Tannins act like a Velcro strip attaching itself to the iron. This prevents the iron from being absorbed into the blood. And if the iron does not get into the blood it will be of little use to the body.

American Journal of Clinical Nutrition 66(1):168–176, 1997

Try These Other Iron-Rich Recipes

CHAPTER EIGHT

Trimming the Fat

Americans Still Have a Lot to Learn

Unless you are Rumplestiltskin, you probably have a good inkling that too much fat in the diet is not good. And while on paper it appears that as a nation we are improving in the fat intake department, it's not really so!

Here's the part that looks good—the percentage of calories from fat has decreased from about 37 percent in the early 1970s to 34 percent in men and 33 percent in women in the 1990s. So what's the worry? During that time period calories have increased by three hundred per day for both men and women, and the actual fat grams have *risen,* up by about 3 grams for men and 6 grams for women! Therefore, the "apparent" decrease in the proportion in fat calories is simply because we've shifted overall calories to a higher level; it's not due to lower overall fat gram intake. That would be like throwing a bag of sugar on top of a typical fast food meal of fries and a burger, and saying that you've lowered your fat intake. You may have lowered the percent of calories in fat (because the sugar is 100 percent fat free), but you have not changed fat consumption one iota!

We still have a fat intake problem. Let's take a quick look at why it is so important to watch our fat intake.

DISEASE PREVENTION

Most of the major chronic diseases are related to eating too much fat in the diet.

Heart Disease. The key fat related to heart disease is eating too much saturated fat. Saturated fat in a nutshell is artery-clogging fat; it has the strongest effect on raising the deadliest cholesterol, LDL cholesterol, also known as "bad" cholesterol. Trans fats are also entering the picture as cholesterol raisers. Anywhere that you find hydrogenated fats you will find trans fats, such as margarine, shortening, and baked goods.

Cancer. High-fat diets have been associated with an increase in the risk of cancers of the colon and rectum, prostate, and endometrium. The association between high-fat diets and the risk of breast cancer is much weaker, but it may play a role through its direct effect on increased blood estrogen levels.

Obesity. This has become a sticky issue. High-fat diets have been related to obesity, which was thought to be due in part to the fact that fat has twice the calories of protein and carbohydrates. But now with an abundance of fat-free foods, it's possible to overconsume calories without a high fat diet. In fact, one scientist recently remarked, "The low-fat products now available are not quite what scientists had in mind when guidelines for low-fat high-carbohydrates were formulated." Indeed! We now have fat-free fat, fat-free ice cream, fat-free cake—so it's all too easy to get fat without eating a speck of fat grams. Our nation's girth has expanded. The prevalence of overweight adults has increased from one quarter of our nation in the early 1970s to one third of Americans in the 1990s.

BEWARE OF FAT-FREE EXTREMISM—WE DO NEED SOME FAT IN THE DIET

Despite fat's bad reputation, it is possible to fall short of this nutrient. Long before fat-free mania, it was commonly thought that it would be difficult to eat a diet too low in fat. But with the advent of highly refined fat-free foods from fat-free margarine to fat-free chips, it's now a real possibility. Low-fat diets not based on whole foods are low in essential fatty acids. Researchers at Boston University Medical Center Hospital have been tracking such a problem. They have found that essential fatty acid insufficiency is one of the most prevalent nutritional deficiencies occurring in the Framingham Offspring Study (not yet published).

Our body requires two essential fatty acids, linoleic and linolenic acid, just like vitamins. Like essential vitamins, essential fatty acids cannot be made sufficiently by the body and must be supplied by the diet. Signs of getting inadequate amounts of these fat nutrients include scaling skin, hair falling out, and problems healing. Good sources of essential fatty acids are nuts, seeds, green leafy vegetables, and vegetable oils (except olive oil is not a good source). We only need a few grams (about one teaspoon) of essential fatty acids a day. While this number is very small, it may be tough to achieve when one is eschewing fat.

Other Roles of Fat. Fat in the diet is also important because it helps the body absorb the fat-soluble vitamins A, D, E, and K. Fat also plays an important role in satisfying hunger. That's why some people are hungry within an hour or two after eating a very low-fat meal. But fat's satiety role is a double-edged sword. The caveat is this: Research shows that fat initially has a weak effect on satiety, which could lead to "passive overeating" if your meal is made up of mainly fatty foods. But once fat reaches your intestine it does generate a potent satiety signal. That's why it is important to have the right balance of foods at meals.

BY THE NUMBERS—HOW MUCH FAT?

Most health authorities, from the American Heart Association to the United States government, recommend that we eat no more than 30 percent of our total calories as fat. Research will most likely refine that number, but for now it's a good place to start. Here's what 30 percent of fat calories looks like in terms of grams of fat.

CALORIES EATEN	MAXIMUM FAT GRAMS (30% fat calories)
1500	50
1600	53
1700	60
1800	60
1900	63
2000	67

Calories Eaten	Maximum Fat Grams (30% fat calories)
2100	70
2200	73
2300	77
2400	80
2500	83
3000	100

CUTTING THE FAT (WHERE YOU WON'T MISS IT)

When it comes to cutting the fat in my recipes I have three principles:

1. *Discover how you can cut the fat without missing it or feeling deprived.* I've met many people who get a little too enthusiastic, to the point that they try taking the fat out of everything only to wind up deflated when the recipe doesn't taste quite right. It's best to start out trying one fat-cutting technique at a time and build on your success. Some of my favorite examples are using fruit purees such as applesauce when baking cakes, brownies, and muffins. Or switching to reduced-fat dairy products. For example, I am fond of using reduced-fat cheese, but find that in most cases fat-free varieties have little to be desired in flavor and texture.

   Be judicious when using fat-free products; they can be a healthy adjunct, but they don't always work the same way as their regular counterparts in a recipe. Many fat-free products have extra water and gelatin, and when baked can turn into a watery mess. Check out Twenty Ways to Trim the Fat from Your Diet, page 201, for more ideas.

2. *When possible choose healthier fats.* The healthiest fats are low in saturated fat and include these oils: canola, corn, olive, safflower, and sunflower oil.

3. *When you eat fat, make sure it's worth it.* When I eat fat, I want to taste every gram! That's why I'm fond of strong-flavored fats such as sesame oil, toasted nuts, and, yes, even a judicious use of butter. On the other hand, it is important to watch out for redundant

use of fat, such as preparing tuna salad with mayonnaise and then slathering the bread with it.

Five Ways to Trim the Fat from Meals

1. Crisp it up—instead of deep frying, try a three-layer coating. First dredge in flour, dip in an egg white wash, and add a crunchy coating like cornflake crumbs. The Onion Rings, page 214, are a great example.

2. Egg whites—use two egg whites for each whole egg. You'll get rid of a lot of cholesterol and save 5 grams of fat for each whole egg replaced. Try the Denver Omelet, page 218, for a delicious example.

3. Use a leaner cut of meat—for example, pork tenderloin is the leanest cut of pork, with a nutrition profile comparable to chicken. Try the Sweet and Sour Pork, page 211.

4. Fruit purees instead of fat—this is a tried and true method, used in place of all or part of the fat in baked goods such as the Lemon-Poppyseed Muffins, page 220. The most readily available fruit puree is good old applesauce.

5. Dry fry—many recipes with meat and chicken call for pan-frying in oil. Instead, try cooking with a little nonstick vegetable oil such as in Savory Breaded Turkey Cutlets, page 205.

Fat Lexicon

✕ ✕ ✕

Term	Meaning
Cholesterol	A fatlike substance that comes only from animal foods and is also made by our own bodies. Blood cholesterol should be less than 200 mg/dl. Levels of 240 or more are considered high risk. Maximum cholesterol from our diet should not exceed 300 milligrams per day.
Essential Fatty Acids	These fats are like vitamins in that the body cannot make them and they are essential for living. The two essential fatty acids are linoleic and linolenic acid.
HDL Cholesterol	Commonly known as "good" cholesterol because it helps to remove the harmful cholesterol from the blood.
Hydrogenated Fat	This is a fat (usually an oil) to which hydrogen has been added. It makes oil spreadable or firmer. It's commonly found in stick margarine, shortening, and baked goods. It behaves like a saturated fat in terms of its cholesterol-raising effects.
LDL Cholesterol	Commonly known as "bad" cholesterol. This is the cholesterol in the blood that is related to heart disease. Blood levels should be less than 130 mg/dl. A high risk level is 160 mg/dl or more.
Low-Fat Food	A legal term on the food label. Has a maximum of 3 grams of fat per serving unless it is a main dish. Main dish products have no more than 3 grams of fat for each 100 calories and no more than 30 percent of calories from fat.
Saturated Fat	Saturated fat raises cholesterol more than any other dietary factor. Saturated fats are found in fatty animal foods such as whole milk products, regular cheeses, lard, and meats. Other sources include coconut oil, coconut milk, and shortening. Health authorities recommend no more than 10 percent of your calories come from this troublesome fat, which is a maximum 20 grams of saturated fat a day for most people.
Trans Fatty Acids	Trans fatty acids are created when hydrogen is added to an oil—most notably with margarine. The problem with trans fatty acids is that they appear to raise the risk of heart disease because they raise blood cholesterol levels. To keep your trans fatty acids low, use soft or liquid margarine. Watch out for processed foods that contain "hydrogenated oils" such as crackers, cookies, and other baked goods.

Twenty Ways to Trim the Fat from Your Diet

1. Eliminate dabs of butter on casserole toppings.
2. Thicken soups with cornstarch or potatoes instead of cream.
3. Toast nuts such as almonds to bring out their wonderfully nutty flavor and use less of them.
4. Replace oil in marinades with a neutral juice such as white grape juice or apple juice.
5. Remove the skin from chicken before cooking.
6. Use evaporated skim milk in place of cream in casseroles, quiches, and cream soup recipes.
7. Toast corn tortillas in the oven and use them in place of fried tortilla chips.
8. Sauté using broth, wine, or nonstick vegetable spray.
9. Use cocoa powder in place of some or all baking chocolate.
10. Make gravy using broth instead of meat drippings. Thicken with cornstarch.
11. In desserts calling for chocolate chips, reduce the amount and use mini chocolate chips to distribute the chocolate richness.
12. Instead of using a roux (flour and butter) to thicken stews, use a cornstarch paste such as cornstarch and broth or cornstarch and water.
13. Use highly flavored cheese in smaller amounts, such as sharp Cheddar, Feta, and real Parmesan.
14. Try using phyllo dough (with nonstick vegetable spray) instead of a traditional pastry crust in dessert pies and savory pot pies.
15. In graham cracker crusts, use melted apricot jam instead of butter to "glue" the crumbs together.
16. Use nonfat milk instead of regular milk in puddings, casseroles, and soups. For extra richness use evaporated skim milk.
17. Are you a butter lover? Try light butter—it has half the fat and calories and tastes terrific.
18. In frostings try using marshmallow creme for all or part of the butter.
19. Invest in a good set of nonstick cookware for easy low-fat cooking.
20. Many recipes that use ground meat traditionally call for one pound, but there's nothing special about that amount. Use three quarters to half the quantity, especially in casseroles, sauces, and soups. Of course, use the leanest variety.

✳ Thai-Style Peanut Noodle Salad ✳

This aromatic salad bursts with flavor and a variety of textures, from the crunchy nuts to the delicate noodles.

THE SNEAK:

- Peanut butter is used instead of peanut oil.
- Reduce the quantity of peanuts and toast them to enhance flavor.

NUTRITION SCORECARD (PER SERVING)			NOTABLE NUTRIENT (PER SERVING)		
	BEFORE	AFTER			
Calories	521	386			
Fat (grams)	29.8	12.5		AMOUNT	% DAILY VALUE
% Fat calories	50	28			
Protein (grams)	12	14	Vitamin A (RE)	759	76
Carbohydrates			Vitamin C		
(grams)	54	57	(milligrams)	33	56
Cholesterol					
(milligrams)	0	0			

THAI-STYLE DRESSING

- ⅓ cup peanut butter
- ¼ cup seasoned rice vinegar
- 3 tablespoons light soy sauce
- 2 tablespoons sugar
- 2 teaspoons finely minced ginger
- 2 teaspoons sesame oil
- 1 clove garlic, minced
- 1½ teaspoons hot chili sauce
- ¼ teaspoon cayenne

SALAD

- 12 ounces linguini noodles
- 3 tablespoons peanuts, chopped
- 1 cup thinly sliced red cabbage
- 2 carrots, cut matchstick style
- 1 red bell pepper, thinly sliced
- ½ cup chopped chives
- ½ cup chopped cilantro

To make the Thai-Style Dressing: In a small bowl whisk together the peanut butter, vinegar, soy sauce, sugar, ginger, sesame oil, garlic, hot chili sauce, and cayenne.

To make the salad: Cook the noodles according to the manufacturer's directions. Rinse with cold water and drain well. Spread the chopped peanuts on a baking sheet and bake at 350°F for 10 minutes until golden and fragrant. Remove from the oven and set aside.

In a large bowl combine the cooked noodles, red cabbage, carrots, red bell pepper, chives, and cilantro. Add the Thai dressing and toss to coat. Divide among six salad plates. Sprinkle the nuts on top of the salad.

Makes 6 servings

Chicken Salad with Creamy Lime–Cilantro Vinaigrette

If you want to prepare this salad in advance, sprinkle a few drops of the lime juice over the avocado. The vitamin C from the lime will prevent it from turning brown.

THE SNEAK:

- Fat-free sour cream is used in place of oil.
- Tortilla chips are home baked rather than fried.
- The amount of cheese is reduced.

NUTRITION SCORECARD (PER SERVING)

	BEFORE	AFTER
Calories	394	210
Fat (grams)	28.2	6.4
% Fat calories	62	27
Protein (grams)	20	20
Carbohydrates (grams)	18	20
Cholesterol (milligrams)	48	44

NOTABLE NUTRIENT (PER SERVING)

	AMOUNT	% DAILY VALUE
Vitamin C (milligrams)	114	190
Fiber (grams)	5	20

CREAMY LIME–CILANTRO VINAIGRETTE

½ cup fat-free sour cream
¼ cup fresh lime juice (about 2 limes)
¼ cup finely snipped cilantro
4 teaspoons white wine vinegar
3 cloves garlic, minced
1 tablespoon minced shallots
½ teaspoon salt
⅛ teaspoon black pepper

SALAD

3 corn tortillas
4 cups thinly sliced romaine
4 cups thinly sliced napa cabbage
2 cups diced cooked chicken
2 tomatoes, diced
1 red bell pepper, thinly sliced
1 yellow bell pepper, thinly sliced
½ avocado, diced
¼ cup fresh corn kernels, or frozen, thawed
¼ cup thinly sliced red onions
¼ cup crumbled Feta cheese

To make the creamy lime–cilantro vinaigrette: In a small bowl whisk together the fat-free sour cream, lime juice, cilantro, vinegar, garlic, shallots, salt, and pepper. Cover and chill while preparing the salad.

To make the salad: Preheat the oven to 375°F. Spray a baking sheet with nonstick vegetable spray. Cut the tortillas in half and then into short ½-inch strips. Place the tortilla strips in a single layer on the baking sheet. Spray the strips with nonstick spray (this will help them to crisp). Bake for 10 minutes until golden brown.

Meanwhile, in a large bowl combine the romaine, cabbage, chicken, tomatoes, the red bell pepper, the yellow bell pepper, avocado, corn kernels, red onions, and Feta cheese.

When ready to serve, toss the salad with the vinaigrette to coat. Sprinkle with the tortilla strips.

Makes 6 servings

Sales of "healthy" products—those foods and beverages with low fat and low cholesterol—expect to grow to $40 billion by the year 2000.
Calorie Control Council. Trends and statistics. www.caloriecontrol.org, 1997

Savory Breaded Turkey Cutlets ✖

This main dish also makes a great appetizer. Just cut the cooked turkey into wedges and insert a decorative toothpick—it's a hit every time!

THE SNEAK:

- Replaces whole egg with egg whites
- Pan-fry using nonstick vegetable spray instead of butter
- Reduces the amount of cheese

NUTRITION SCORECARD (PER SERVING)	BEFORE	AFTER
Calories	495	339
Fat (grams)	24.9	7.2
% Fat calories	46	25
Protein (grams)	38	34
Carbohydrates (grams)	28	28
Cholesterol (milligrams)	212	65

¼ cup all-purpose flour
¼ teaspoon salt
⅛ teaspoon black pepper
2 egg whites
1 cup seasoned bread crumbs

¼ cup grated Parmesan cheese
4 (3-ounce) turkey breast slices, ¼ inch thick
spaghetti sauce (optional)

In a shallow dish stir together the flour, salt, and pepper. In a second shallow dish lightly beat the egg whites. In a third shallow dish combine the bread crumbs and Parmesan cheese.

Dip each turkey slice first in the flour mixture, next in the egg whites, and then in the bread crumbs to coat.

Spray a large skillet with nonstick vegetable spray. Heat the pan over medium-high heat and add the coated turkey slices. Cook for 2 to 3 minutes on each side until no pink remains. If desired, serve with spaghetti sauce.

Makes 4 servings

✖ Turkey Pot Pie for a Crowd ✖

This is a hearty winner with its elegant crust of phyllo. If you have little or no experience with phyllo dough, this is a good recipe to start with. One sheet nearly fits the pan, so there's not a lot of fussing.

THE SNEAK:

- Phyllo dough is used instead of the traditional pastry crust.
- Margarine is eliminated.
- Replace whole milk with evaporated skim milk.

NUTRITION SCORECARD (PER SERVING)			NOTABLE NUTRIENT (PER SERVING)		
	BEFORE	AFTER			
Calories	685	222			
Fat (grams)	38	1.6		AMOUNT	% DAILY VALUE
% Fat calories	50	7			
Protein (grams)	34	24	Vitamin A (RE)	250	25
Carbohydrates (grams)	47	28			
Cholesterol (milligrams)	110	47			

2 cups diced potatoes
2 cups chopped fresh mushrooms
½ cup chopped onion
¾ teaspoon dried sage leaves
½ teaspoon thyme
½ teaspoon rosemary
¼ teaspoon salt
¼ teaspoon black pepper
2 cups fat-free chicken broth

¾ cup evaporated skim milk
3 tablespoons cornstarch
1 (10-ounce) package frozen mixed vegetables, thawed and drained
3 cups diced cooked turkey breast
¼ cup snipped parsley
5 sheets phyllo dough

Place the diced potatoes on a paper plate and cover with wax paper. Microwave on high for 1 to 2 minutes until tender.

Spray a 4-quart saucepan with nonstick cooking spray. Add the mushrooms and onion. Cook and stir over medium heat until the onion is translucent. Stir in the sage leaves, thyme, rosemary, salt, and black pepper. Add the broth. In a small cup stir together ¼ cup evaporated skim milk and cornstarch until smooth. Add the cornstarch mixture and remaining milk to the onion broth mixture. Cook and stir until thickened and bubbly.

Stir in the potatoes, vegetables, turkey, and parsley. Cook and stir until bubbly. Pour the turkey mixture into a 13 × 9 × 2-inch pan. Preheat the oven to 375°F.

Lay one sheet of the phyllo dough on top of the turkey mixture. Spray the dough with nonstick spray. Crumple the edges of the dough to fit the pan. Repeat layering, spraying, and crumpling with remaining phyllo dough sheets. Bake at 375°F for 15 to 20 minutes until golden.

Makes 8 servings

Source of Trans Fat in the Diet

Vegetable shortening	14–18% trans fat
Tub margarine	11–28% trans fat
Stick margarine	19–49% trans fat

American Journal of Clinical Nutrition 62(3s):657s–658s, 1995

Trans Fats Increase Heart Disease Risk

Recent results from the Nurse's Health Study underscore the problem of trans fats (which act like artery–clogging saturated fat). Diets of over eighty thousand women were examined during a fourteen-year period. Results suggest that by eliminating the trans fats (which represented only about 2 percent of calories in their diet) and replacing it with healthier fats would reduce the risk of heart disease by a whopping 53 percent.

New England Journal of Medicine 337(21):1491–1499, 1997

Tarragon Chicken
✹ with Mushroom Sauce ✹

*Flattening the chicken breasts with a mallet helps to speed up
the cooking time.*

THE SNEAK:

- Eliminating most of the butter and oil for the sauce and cooking
- Pan-frying using nonstick vegetable spray

NUTRITION SCORECARD (PER SERVING)		
	BEFORE	AFTER
Calories	360	216
Fat (grams)	20.1	3.7
% Fat calories	53	15
Protein (grams)	30	30
Carbohydrates (grams)	10	10
Cholesterol (milligrams)	100	73

4	boneless, skinless chicken breasts (about 1 pound)	1	teaspoon olive oil
¼	cup all-purpose flour	¼	cup chopped onion
¾	teaspoon tarragon	½	pound sliced mushrooms
¼	teaspoon salt	½	cup chicken broth
⅛	teaspoon black pepper	½	cup dry white wine
		1	tablespoon light butter

Place each chicken breast between two sheets of heavy-duty plastic wrap
and pound from the center outward with the flat side of a meat mallet or
other heavy utensil until ¼ inch thick.

In a shallow bowl combine the flour, tarragon, salt, and pepper. Dredge
the chicken in the flour mixture to coat, reserving the remaining flour.

Spray a large skillet with nonstick vegetable spray and heat over
medium-high heat. Add the dredged chicken in batches and cook until
browned on each side. Transfer the browned chicken to a shallow baking pan.

Add the olive oil to the hot pan along with the onion and reserved flour. Carefully cook and stir for 1 minute. Add the mushrooms and cook and stir 1 additional minute. Stir in the chicken broth and wine. Bring to a boil, constantly stirring. Whisk the butter into the hot sauce. Remove from the heat. Pour the sauce over the chicken. Bake uncovered for 20 minutes until heated through.

Makes 4 servings

✳ Kung Pao Chicken ✳

This popular Chinese dish is traditionally fried with the skin on. But you won't miss the skin or oil because of its flavorful and spicy sauce. Most grocery stores carry the bean sauce, hoisin sauce, and chili paste in the international or Asian section. This dish pairs up nicely with the Stir-fried Rice on page 160.

THE SNEAK:

- Skin is removed from the chicken.
- Chicken is stir-fried without deep frying.
- Reduce the amount of nuts.

NUTRITION SCORECARD (PER SERVING)		
	BEFORE	**AFTER**
Calories	656	221
Fat (grams)	47.8	6.6
% Fat calories	65	27
Protein (grams)	44	30
Carbohydrates (grams)	15	10
Cholesterol (milligrams)	95	65

Chicken Marinade

- 1 egg white
- 2 teaspoons cornstarch
- 4 boneless, skinless chicken breasts (1 pound)

Kung Pao Sauce

- 2 tablespoons black bean sauce
- 1 tablespoon hoisin sauce
- 1 teaspoon Szechwan chili paste with garlic
- 2 teaspoons sugar
- 1 tablespoon dry sherry
- 1 tablespoon red wine vinegar
- 4 cloves garlic, minced
- 4 tablespoons peanuts
- ½ teaspoon crushed red pepper flakes

To make the chicken marinade: In a medium bowl stir together the egg white and cornstarch until smooth. Cut the chicken into bite-size cubes and toss with the cornstarch mixture to coat. Set aside.

To make the Kung Pao sauce: In a small bowl combine the bean sauce, hoisin, chili paste, sugar, sherry, vinegar, and garlic.

To prepare the dish, spray a wok or large skillet with nonstick spray. Add the peanuts and crushed red pepper. Cook and stir over medium-high heat until golden. Remove and set aside. Add the chicken with its marinade. Cook and stir until cooked through and no longer pink, about 5 minutes. Add the sauce and cook until heated through; serve.

Makes 4 servings

Sweet and Sour Pork

Traditionally the meat in this recipe is fried, but because of the ample sauce it's bathed in, most people are not aware of this fatty fact. Even without frying, this saucy dish is so delicious you'll be licking your plate clean. Note: This recipe also works with chicken breasts.

THE SNEAK:

- Uses pork tenderloin—the leanest cut of pork
- Replaces whole egg with egg white
- Eliminates frying and instead uses nonstick vegetable spray

NUTRITION SCORECARD (PER SERVING)			NOTABLE NUTRIENT (PER SERVING)		
	BEFORE	AFTER			
Calories	493	379			
Fat (grams)	16	3.9		AMOUNT	% DAILY VALUE
% Fat calories	11	9			
Protein (grams)	17	22	Vitamin A (RE)	708	71
Carbohydrates			Vitamin C	27	46
(grams)	74	66	(milligrams)		
Cholesterol					
(milligrams)	70	45			

MEAT MARINADE

1 tablespoon all-purpose flour
1 tablespoon cornstarch
½ teaspoon salt
¼ teaspoon pepper

2 egg whites
1 pound pork tenderloin, cut into ¾-inch cubes

Sweet and Sour Sauce

¼ cup sugar
2 tablespoons cornstarch
⅛ teaspoon cinnamon
1 (20-ounce) can pineapple tidbits, packed in juice (reserve juice)
¾ cup water
⅓ cup rice vinegar
½ cup catsup
1 tablespoon light soy sauce

Stir-fry Mixture

1 cup chopped onions
2 medium carrots, cut matchstick style into 1-inch strips
1 green bell pepper, cut into ½-inch squares
1 clove garlic, minced
6 shiitake mushrooms, sliced (if dried, soak according to package directions)
3 cups hot cooked brown rice

To make the meat marinade: In a small bowl stir together the flour, cornstarch, salt, and pepper. Add the egg whites, stirring until smooth. Add the pork cubes, stirring to coat.

To make the sweet and sour sauce: In a 4-quart saucepan stir together the sugar, cornstarch, and cinnamon. Drain the pineapple, reserving ¾ cup of juice, and stir into the cornstarch mixture (pineapple will be used later). Stir in the water, rice vinegar, catsup, and soy sauce. Cook and stir over medium heat until thickened and bubbly, about 10 minutes. Cook and stir for 1 minute more. Reduce the heat to the lowest setting and cover.

To make the stir-fry mixture: Spray a wok or large skillet with non-stick spray. Over medium-high heat cook and stir the onions, carrots, bell pepper, and garlic for 3 minutes. Add the mushrooms and cook for 1 additional minute. Using a slotted spoon mix the vegetables into the sweet and sour sauce. Add the pork mixture to the wok and cook and stir until no longer pink, about 5 to 7 minutes. Transfer to the sweet and sour mixture. Stir in pineapple. Serve over brown rice.

Makes 6 servings

❋ Garlic Mashed Potatoes ❋

These mashed potatoes can satisfy like nothing else. Red potatoes impart a creamier texture than traditional russet potatoes, which are mealy. To help retain valuable vitamins and minerals, I recommend cooking the potatoes with their skins on. Otherwise, it's all too easy for the nutrients to get leached out into the water.

THE SNEAK:

- Nonfat milk is used instead of heavy cream.
- Olive oil is eliminated.
- Butter is replaced with light butter, and much less of it.

NUTRITION SCORECARD (PER SERVING)		
	BEFORE	**AFTER**
Calories	339	186
Fat (grams)	18.8	1.2
% Fat calories	49	5
Protein (grams)	4	4
Carbohydrates (grams)	41	41
Cholesterol (milligrams)	28	3

3	pounds red potatoes, washed	1	tablespoon light butter
¼	cup skim milk	¾	teaspoon salt
3	cloves garlic, minced	¼	teaspoon black pepper

Fill a saucepan three quarters full with water and bring to a boil. Add the potatoes and boil until fork tender, about 40 minutes.

Drain the potatoes. Carefully peel and return to the pan. Place over low heat and using a potato masher, mash the potatoes while mixing in half of the milk, garlic, butter, salt, and pepper. Slowly add the remaining milk until at the desired consistency. Serve immediately.

Makes 6 servings

✖ Onion Rings (Practically Fat Free) ✖

It's no secret that frying adds lots of fat, but when food (in this case, onion rings) is coated in flour or a breading, even more fat is absorbed! Since these rings are oven-baked there is no problem with fat.

THE SNEAK:

- Baking instead of frying
- Adding a coating of cornflake crumbs for extra crunchiness
- A spritz of nonstick spray on the coated onions enhances crispness.

NUTRITION SCORECARD (PER SERVING)			
	BEFORE	AFTER	
Calories	550	245	
Fat (grams)	47	0.4	
% Fat calories	77	1	
Protein (grams)	7	9	
Carbohydrates (grams)	26	52	
Cholesterol (milligrams)	0	0	

3	large onions, sliced ¼ inch thick	1	teaspoon paprika
1	cup buttermilk	½	teaspoon salt
½	cup all-purpose flour	4	egg whites
		1½	cups cornflake crumbs

Separate the onions into rings and mix with the buttermilk in a large bowl to coat. Stir occasionally and set aside for at least 20 minutes.

Preheat the oven to 375°F. Spray a baking sheet with nonstick vegetable spray.

In a shallow dish stir together the flour, paprika, and salt. In a second shallow dish lightly beat the egg whites. In a third shallow dish add the cornflake crumbs.

Dip each onion ring first in the flour mixture, next in the egg whites, and then in the cornflake crumbs to coat. Place on the prepared baking sheet. Spray the onion rings with nonstick spray. Bake in batches for 15 minutes until golden. Serve immediately.

Makes 4 servings

Polenta with Fresh Corn

This is one polenta dish that you won't have to labor over, stirring and stirring. The fresh corn with a bit of onion makes it particularly enjoyable. Chilling the polenta overnight and then broiling provides a nice firm texture.

THE SNEAK:

- Light butter (and less of it) is used instead of butter.
- Use reduced-fat cheese.

NUTRITION SCORECARD (PER SERVING)

	BEFORE	AFTER
Calories	222	172
Fat (grams)	9.6	3.6
% Fat calories	38	18
Protein (grams)	6	7
Carbohydrates (grams)	30	30
Cholesterol (milligrams)	24	9

1 tablespoon light butter
2 cups fresh yellow corn (2 ears)
1/4 cup chopped onion
1 cup cornmeal
2 teaspoons sugar
3/4 teaspoon salt
3 cups water
1/2 cup shredded reduced-fat sharp Cheddar cheese

In a large microwave-safe dish add the butter, corn, and onion. Microwave on High, stirring occasionally until the onion is transparent, about 2 minutes.

Stir in the cornmeal, sugar, salt, and water. Microwave on High for 4 minutes, stirring every minute to smooth out any lumps. Cook until the mixture is very thick and somewhat pourable, about 4 minutes, stirring occasionally.

Spray a 1½- or 2-quart loaf pan with nonstick spray. Transfer the polenta to a loaf pan and cover with plastic wrap. Cover and chill overnight for at least 6 hours until firm.

Preheat the broiler. Spray a baking sheet with nonstick spray. Remove the plastic wrap from the loaf pan and slip a knife around the edges to free the polenta. Unmold onto a cutting board, tapping sharply to release if necessary.

Cut the polenta into ¾-inch slices and arrange in a single layer on a prepared baking sheet. Broil 3 to 4 inches from the heat until the polenta begins to form a golden crust, about 5 minutes. Turn the polenta with a spatula and broil on the second side until golden, 4 to 5 minutes longer. Turn off the broiler, top the polenta with cheese, and return to the oven until the cheese melts, about 1 minute.

Makes 6 servings

Ultra Low-Fat Diet May Be of No Benefit

Volunteers (444 men) with high cholesterol were given one of four fat-modified diets for a period of one year. The dietary fat levels ranged from 18 to 30 percent of total calories. The men with the highest cholesterol saw the most dramatic drop in LDL (bad cholesterol) with the least restrictive of the four regimens—30 percent fat calorie diet. The other diets were found not only to be without added benefit in terms of cholesterol reduction but they decreased the protective HDL or "good" cholesterol.

Journal of the American Medical Association (18):1509–1515, 1997

Easy Brunch Casserole

It's hard to believe that this sophisticated-looking dish is so simple to make. The texture resembles a delicate soufflé, but the beauty is that you prepare everything the night before. When guests arrive, you merely pop this dish into the oven.

THE SNEAK:

- Egg whites are used instead of whole eggs, and the dried mustard powder provides a nice yellow color.
- A combination of evaporated nonfat milk and regular nonfat milk is used instead of whole milk.
- Lean turkey sausage is used in place of regular sausage.
- Reduced-fat cheese is used instead of regular cheese.

NUTRITION SCORECARD (PER SERVING)

	BEFORE	AFTER
Calories	717	284
Fat (grams)	49.7	9.1
% Fat calories	63	29
Protein (grams)	41	23
Carbohydrates (grams)	25	26
Cholesterol (milligrams)	408	103

NOTABLE NUTRIENT (PER SERVING)

	AMOUNT	% DAILY VALUE
Calcium (milligrams)	387	39

- ½ chopped onion
- 2 (3-ounce) lean turkey sausage links, casings removed
- 4 egg whites
- 2 whole large eggs
- 1½ cups nonfat evaporated milk
- ¼ cup regular nonfat milk
- 2 teaspoons dry mustard
- ¼ teaspoon salt
- ⅛ teaspoon pepper
- 7 slices firm buttermilk or sourdough bread, crusts trimmed
- ½ cup shredded reduced-fat (not fat-free) Cheddar cheese
- ½ cup shredded reduced-fat (not fat-free) Monterey Jack cheese

Spray a nonstick large skillet with nonstick vegetable spray. Cook the onion and turkey sausage over medium heat until the sausage is cooked through. While stirring the sausage, crumble into small pieces. Set aside.

Meanwhile, in a large bowl beat together the egg whites, whole eggs, nonfat evaporated milk, regular nonfat milk, dry mustard, salt, and pepper.

Lightly spray a 9-inch deep dish pie plate with nonstick vegetable spray. Slice the bread diagonally, into quarters, making four triangles for each slice. Arrange half of the bread pieces in a single layer in the pie dish. Add another layer of the remaining bread pieces. Top with the sausage-onion mixture. Sprinkle the cheeses over the sausage. Pour the egg mixture over all. Cover and refrigerate overnight.

Preheat the oven to 350°F. Uncover the dish and bake for about 45 minutes until golden and puffy. Serve immediately.

Makes 6 servings

✳ Denver Omelet ✳

While you can certainly make an omelet with just egg whites or egg substitutes, I prefer the ratio of 1 whole egg to 2 egg whites. It lends a nicer, less rubbery texture and a richer yellow color.

THE SNEAK:

- Uses two egg whites for one of the whole eggs
- Eliminates butter
- Uses turkey ham in place of regular ham and bacon
- Bonus sneak: It's not too often that people get a chance to eat vegetables with breakfast. An omelet is a great vehicle for delivering the greens, in this case, bell pepper.

NUTRITION SCORECARD (PER SERVING)			NOTABLE NUTRIENT (PER SERVING)		
	BEFORE	AFTER			
Calories	445	166			
Fat (grams)	36.3	6.6		AMOUNT	% DAILY VALUE
% Fat calories	74	36			
Protein (grams)	22	19	Vitamin C		
Carbohydrates			(milligrams)	25	42
(grams)	6	6			
Cholesterol					
(milligrams)	482	229			

2	egg whites	¼	cup diced green bell pepper
1	whole egg	¼	cup diced onion
⅛	teaspoon salt	1	piece (1 ounce) turkey ham,
	dash of black pepper		diced

In a small bowl beat together the egg whites, whole egg, salt, and black pepper.

Spray a small nonstick omelet pan or small skillet with nonstick vegetable spray. Add the bell pepper, onion, and turkey ham. Cook and stir over medium heat until the onion is translucent.

Add the egg mixture and cook *without* stirring until the omelet begins to set around the edges, about 10 seconds. Then using a rubber spatula, lift the edges of the cooked portion of the omelet to let the uncooked egg mixture flow under it. Repeat until most of the omelet is set. Cover the pan with a lid and cook for 30 to 45 seconds more until the eggs are cooked to desired doneness.

Slide the omelet halfway onto a plate, then flip it over itself.

Makes 1 serving

✺ Lemon-Poppyseed Muffins ✺

*These muffins are accented with fresh lemon peel and make for a great
snack served with a spot of your favorite herbal tea. Don't forget to
grate the lemon peel before you juice the lemons!*

THE SNEAK:

- Egg whites are used in place of whole eggs.
- Applesauce is used instead of butter.
- Fat-free sour cream is used instead of its regular counterpart.
- The bonus sneak is whole wheat flour, which is incorporated with the
  all-purpose flour. This is especially easy to pull off with the added tex-
  ture of the poppyseeds.

NUTRITION SCORECARD (PER MUFFIN)		
	BEFORE	AFTER
Calories	239	152
Fat (grams)	12.0	1.2
% Fat calories	44	7
Protein (grams)	4	4
Carbohydrates (grams)	30	32
Cholesterol (milligrams)	61	0

1	cup all-purpose flour	½	cup fat-free sour cream
½	cup whole wheat flour	½	cup applesauce
1	cup sugar	2	tablespoons fresh lemon juice
3	tablespoons poppyseeds	1	tablespoon finely grated
2	teaspoons baking powder		lemon peel (zest)
½	teaspoon salt	1	tablespoon powdered sugar
3	egg whites		

Spray a standard 12-cup muffin tin with nonstick vegetable spray. Preheat
the oven to 400°F.

In a large bowl combine all of the dry ingredients: all-purpose flour,
whole wheat flour, sugar, poppyseeds, baking powder, and salt.

In a medium bowl beat the egg whites until foamy. Stir in the fat-free sour cream, applesauce, lemon juice, and lemon peel until thoroughly combined. Add the egg white mixture all at once to the flour mixture. Stir just until moistened.

Divide the batter evenly into the muffin tin (filling each until nearly full). Bake for 18 to 22 minutes until golden. When cool remove from the pan. Sprinkle with powdered sugar.

Makes 12 muffins

High-Fat Foods Least Satiating . . . Could Lead to Overeating

Researchers from the University of Sydney, Australia, created the first validated satiety index of common foods. (Note, satiation controls meal size while satiety measures the capacity of food to control subsequent hunger.) People were fed the same number of calories from thirty-eight different foods. (For example, 240 calories of peanuts and 240 calories of potatoes and so on.) The volunteers rated their satiety level every fifteen minutes over a two-hour period.

Researchers found that the foods highest in fat were the least satiating and suggest that the early satiating capacity of food strongly influences how much you will eat at a meal or within the next few hours if an opportunity to eat arises.

Foods that were the most filling? Those highest in fiber. For example, whole wheat bread was more satisfying than white bread, whole wheat pasta scored higher than white pasta.

European Journal of Clinical Nutrition 49(9):675–690, 1995

✖ Dried Cherry Strudel Turnovers ✖

Don't be intimidated by phyllo dough; it's a great asset for low-fat cooking, especially in pastries and pastry crusts. It's very simple to use—if you tear a piece, just grab another. Toasted almonds make this dried cherry filling irresistible.

THE SNEAK:

- Nonstick vegetable spray is used instead of butter for the phyllo sheets.
- The amount of almonds is reduced, but the almonds are toasted to bring out their rich and nutty flavor.

NUTRITION SCORECARD (PER SERVING)		
	BEFORE	AFTER
Calories	389	250
Fat (grams)	21.6	7.2
% Fat calories	44	22
Protein (grams)	6	5
Carbohydrates (grams)	55	53
Cholesterol (milligrams)	31	0

1	cup dried cherries	6	phyllo sheets, thawed
¾	cup water	4	tablespoons apricot jam,
½	cup slivered almonds		melted
2	tablespoons brown sugar		powdered sugar
1	teaspoon almond extract		

Place the cherries in a small saucepan and add the water. Bring to a boil. Cover, remove from the heat, and let stand for 30 minutes.

Meanwhile, preheat the oven to 350°F. Place the slivered almonds on a baking sheet. Bake for 5 to 7 minutes until golden and fragrant. Remove from the oven and let cool for 10 minutes. Grind the almonds in a food processor or blender until finely chopped. Add the soaked dried cherries and 1 tablespoon of the soaking liquid; discard the remaining liquid. Pulse until coarsely chopped. Add the brown sugar and almond extract. Pulse again until mixed.

To assemble the turnovers: Lightly spray a baking sheet with nonstick vegetable spray.

Place one sheet of the phyllo dough on a large piece of wax paper. (Keep the remaining phyllo sheets covered with a damp cloth to prevent drying out.) Spray the phyllo sheet with nonstick spray. Fold it lengthwise. Add 2 teaspoons of melted jam and spread evenly over the phyllo to ½ inch of the borders. Spoon a mound (about 3 tablespoons) of the dried cherry-almond mixture and place it about 1 inch from one end of the folded phyllo strip. Fold the end over the cherry mixture at a 45° angle. Continue folding to form a triangle that encloses the apple mixture (this is like folding a flag).

Place the turnover on the prepared baking sheet and repeat the procedure with the remaining phyllo dough to make a total of 6 turnovers. Bake for 15 minutes at 350°F for 10 to 15 minutes until golden.

Remove from the oven and transfer to a serving dish. Cut each turnover in half to reveal the filling. Sprinkle with sifted powdered sugar. Serve immediately.

Makes 6 servings, 1 turnover each (2 triangles)

Don't Count on Fake Fat as Weight Loss Aid

Studies in both children and adults show that when part of the fat in the diet is replaced by Olestra, there's a tendency to compensate by eating more of other foods. This compensation effect is more pronounced when fat is lowered to 20 percent of calories.

American Journal of Clinical Nutrition 63(6):891–896, 1996

INTRODUCTION

Birch, L. L. Children's food acceptance patterns. *Nutrition Today* 31(6):234–240, 1996.

Craig, W. J. Phytochemicals: guardians of our health. *Journal of the American Dietetic Association* 97(suppl 2):s199–s204, 1997.

Heaney, R. Food: what a surprise! *American Journal of Clinical Nutrition* 64(5): 791–792, 1996.

Hess, M. A. Taste: the neglected nutritional factor. *Journal of the American Dietetic Association* 97(suppl 2):s205–s207, 1997.

VEGETABLES

Beecher, C.W. W. Cancer preventive properties of varieties of Brassica oleracea: a review. *American Journal of Clinical Nutrition* 59(supplement):1166s–1170s, 1994.

Birch, L. L. Children's food acceptance patterns. *Nutrition Today* 31(6):234–240, 1996.

Block, G. et al. Fruit, vegetables and cancer prevention: a review of the epidemiological evidence. *Nutrition and Cancer* 18:1–29, 1992.

Cao, G. et al. Antioxidant capacity of tea and common vegetables. *Journal of Agricultural and Food Chemistry* 44(22):3426–3431, 1996.

Carver, G. W. *How the Farmer Can Save His Sweet Potatoes and Ways of Preparing them for the Table*. Tuskegee Institute Press: Alabama, November 1936.

Drewnoski, A. From asparagus to zucchini: mapping cognitive space for vegetable names. *Journal of the American College of Nutrition* 15(2):147–153, 1996.

Forman, A. As beta-carotene fades, focus turns to other carotenoids. *Environmental Nutrition* 20(8):4, 1997.

Michnovicz, J. J. et al. Changes in levels of urinary estrogen metabolites after oral indole-3-carbinol treatment in humans. *Journal National Cancer Institute* 89(10) 718–723, 1997.

Report card for Americans' Eating Habits. *Tufts University Health & Nutrition Letter* 15(4):1, 1997.

Schardt, D. Phytochemicals: Plants against cancer. *Nutrition Action Health Letter* 21(3):1, 1994.

Smith, S. et al. The University of Minnesota Cancer Prevention Research Unit vegetable and fruit classification scheme (United States). *Cancer Causes and Control* 6:292–302, 1995.

Steinmetz, K. Vegetables, fruit and cancer prevention: A review. *Journal of the American Dietetic Association* 96:1027–1039, 1996.

FRUIT

Aldoori, W. H. et al. Prospective study of diet and the risk of duodenal ulcer in men. *American Journal of Epidemiology* Jan 1; 145(1):42–50, 1997.

Cook, D. G. Effect of fresh fruit consumption on lung function and wheeze in children. *Thorax* 52(July):628–633.

Dennison, B. A. et al. Excess fruit juice consumption by preschool-aged children is associated with short stature and obesity. *Pediatrics* 99(Jan):15–22, 1997.

Dennison, B. A. Fruit juice consumption by infants and children: a review. *Journal of the American College of Nutrition* 15(Oct):4s–11s, 1996.

Heimendinger, J., and M. A. Van Duyn. Dietary behavior change: the challenge of recasting the role of fruit and vegetables in the American diet. *American Journal of Clinical Nutrition* 61(suppl):1397s–1401s, 1995.

Jang, M. et al. Cancer chemopreventive activity of resveratrol, a natural product derived from grapes. *Science* 275(January 10):218–229, 1997.

Neumark-Sztainer, D. et al. Correlates of inadequate fruit and vegetable consumption among adolescents. *Preventive Medicine* 25(Sept/Oct):497–505, 1996.

Singh, R. B. et al. Can guava fruit intake decrease blood pressure and blood lipids? *Journal Human Hypertension* 7(Feb 3):33–38, 1993.

CALCIUM

Alberston, A. M. et al. Estimated dietary calcium intake and food sources for adolescent females: 1980–92. *Journal Adolescent Health* 20(Jan):20–26, 1997.

Bucher, H. C. et al. Effect of calcium supplementation on pregnancy-induced hypertension and preeclamsia. *Journal of the American Medical Association* 275 (April 10):1113–1117, 1996.

Bucher, H. C. et al. Effect of dietary calcium supplementation on blood pressure—a meta-analysis of randomized controlled trials. *Journal of the American Medical Association* 275(April 3):1016–1022, 1996.

Burros, M. Limiting lead in calcium supplements. *New York Times online.* June 17, 1997.

Curhan, G. C. et al. Comparison of dietary calcium and supplemental calcium and other nutrients as factors affecting the risk of kidney stones in women. *Annals of Internal Medicine* 126:497–504, 1997.

Durgam, V. R. and G. Fernandes. The growth inhibitory effect of conjugated linoleic acid on MCF-7 cells is related to estrogen response system. *Cancer Letter* 116 (June 24):121–130, 1997.

Evans, C. E. et al. The effect of dietary sodium on calcium metabolism in premenopausal and postmenopausal women. *European Journal of Clinical Nutrition* 51(June):394–399, 1997.

Farley, D. Bone Builders. *FDA Consumer* 31(6):27–30, 1997.

Food and Nutrition Board/Institute of Medicine. *Dietary Reference Intakes: Calcium, Phosphorous, Magnesium, Vitamin D, and Fluoride.* Washington, D.C.: National Academy Press, 1997.

Forman, A. Beyond Calcium: Nutrition Strategies to Protect Your Bones. *Environmental Nutrition* 19(December):1, 6, 1996.

Ghadirian, P. et al. Nutritional Factors and Colon Carcinoma. *Cancer* 80:858–864, 1997.

Ip., C. et al. Conjugated linoleic acid. A powerful anticarcinogen. *Cancer* 74 (August 1):1050–1054, 1994.

Lactose irony: the problem may now be the cure. *Environmental Nutrition* 19 (December):3, 1996.

Lin, H. et al. Survey of the conjugated linoleic acid contests of dairy products. *Journal of Dairy Science* 78(Nov):2358–2365, 1995.

Lloyd, T. et al. Dietary caffeine intake and bone status of postmenopausal women. *American Journal of Clinical Nutrition* 65(June):1826–1830, 1997.

National Osteoporosis Foundation. Researchers cite advances in osteoporosis at meeting of international experts. *Cutting Edge Reports Online*, June 1997.

Nieves, J. W. et al. Calcium potentiates the effect of estrogen and calcitonin on bone mass: review and analysis. *American Journal of Clinical Nutrition* 67(1):18–24, 1998.

Optimal Calcium Intake. *NIH Consensus Statement.* June 6–8:12(4):1–31, 1994.

SOY

Anderson, J. W. et al. Meta-analysis of the effects of soy protein intake on serum lipids. *New England Journal of Medicine* (August 3): 333(5):276, 1995.

Arjmandi, B. H. et al. Dietary soybean protein prevents bone loss in an ovariectomized rat model of osteoporosis. *Journal of Nutrition* 126(1):161–167, 1996.

Craig, W. J. Phytochemicals: Guardians of our health. *Journal American Dietetic Association* 97(10 supplement 2):s199–s204, 1997.

Dwyer, J. T. et al. Tofu and soy drinks contain phytoestrogens. *Journal American Dietetic Association* 94(July):739–743, 1994.

Erdman, J. W. Control of serum lipids with soy protein (editorial) *New England Journal of Medicine* (August 3): 333(5):313, 1995.

Goodman, M. T. et al. Association of soy and fiber consumption with the risk of endometrial cancer. *American Journal of Epidemiology* 146(Aug 15):294–306, 1997.

Meisler, J. G. Soy: the bean most likely to suceed in fending off cancer, heart disease. *Environmental Nutrition* 17(5):1, 4, 1994.

Messina, V. and M. Messina. *The Vegetarian Way*. Crown trade paperbacks: NY, 1996.

Potter, S. M. Consumption of isolated soy protein with elevated isoflavones increases spinal bone mass in postmenopausal women. (In submission, and described by researcher in: Erdman, J. W. and S. M. Potter in the *Soy Connection* 5(2):1, 1997.

Research News. Soy in a.m. may relieve sweats in p.m. *Environmental Nutrition* 20(2):8, 1997.

BEANS

Alpert, J. E. and M. Fava. Nutrition and depression: The role of folate. *Nutrition Reviews* 55(5):145–149, 1997.

Anderson, J. W. Serum lipid response of hypercholesterolemic men to single and divided doses of canned beans. *American Journal of Clinical Nutrition* 51(6): 1013–1019, 1990.

Fruhbeck, G. et al. Hormonal implications of the hypocholesterolemic effect of intake of field beans (Vicia faba L.) by young men with hypercholesterolemia. *American Journal of Clinical Nutrition* 66(6):1452–1460, 1997.

Graham, I. et al. Plasma homocysteine as a risk factor for vascular disease: the European concerted action project. *Journal of the American Medical Association* 277(22):1775–1781, 1997.

Hughes, J. S. Dry beans inhibit Azoxymethane-induced colon carcinogenesis in F344 rats. *Journal of Nutrition* 127(12):2328–2333, 1997.

USDA-AGS. Folate deficiency rapidly raises risk. *Food & Nutrition Research Briefs*, April 1, 1996.

USDA-AGS. Folate spares colon and heart. *Food & Nutrition Research Briefs*, July 1, 1996.

FIBER

Anderson, J. W. et al. Health benefits and practical aspects of high-fiber diets. *American Journal of Clinical Nutrition* 59(supplement):1242s–1427s, 1994.

Baer, D. et al. Dietary fiber decreases the metabolizable energy content and nutrient digestibility of mixed diets fed to humans. *Journal of Nutrition* 127(4):579–586, 1997.

Liebman, B. The whole grain guide. *Nutrition Action Health Letter* 24(2):1–11, 1997.

Pietinen, P. et al. Intake of dietary fiber and risk of coronary heart disease in a cohort of Finnish Men: the alpha-tocopherol, beta-carotene cancer prevention study. *Circulation* 94(11):2720–2727, 1996.

Position of the American Dietetic Association: health implications of dietary fiber. *Journal of the American Dietetic Association* 97(10):1157–1159, 1997.

Salmeron, J. et al. Dietary Fiber, glycemic load, and risk of non-insulin dependent Diabetes Mellitus in Women. *Journal of the American Medical Association* 277(6):427–477, 1997.

Slavin, J. L. Whole grains and health: separating the wheat from the chaff. *Nutrition Today* 29(4):6–11, 1994.

The State of America's Plate. Wheat Foods Council: Englewood, CO, 1997.

Tribole, E. The Truth About Fiber. *Consumers Digest*, May/June, 1991.

USDA-AGS. Counting Calories More Precisely. *Food and Nutrition Research Briefs*, July 1997.

IRON

Bruner, A. et al. Randomized study of cognitive effects of iron supplementation in non-anaemic iron-deficient adolescent girls. *Lancet* 348:992–996, 1996.

Dallman, P. R. Biochemical basis for the manifestation of iron deficiency. *Annual Review of Nutrition* 6:13–40, 1986.

Dewey, K. G. et al. Effects of discontinuing coffee intake on iron status of iron-deficient Guatemalan toddlers: a randomized intervention study. *American Journal of Clinical Nutrition* 66(1):168–176, 1997.

Hallberg, L. Search for nutritional confounding factors in the relationship between iron deficiency and brain function. *American Journal of Clinical Nutrition* 50(supplement):598–606, 1989.

Iron's link to heart disease weakened. *Tufts University Health & Nutrition Letter*. 15(3):3, 1997.

Looker, A. C. Prevalence of Iron Deficiency in the United States. *Journal of the American Medical Association* 277(12):973–976, 1997.

National Research Council. *Recommended Dietary Allowances* (10th edition). National Academy Press: Washington, D.C., 1989.

Park J. and H. C. Brittin. Increased iron content of food due to stainless steel cookware. *Journal of the American Dietetic Association* 97(6):659–661, 1997.

Pollitt, E., ed. International conference on iron deficiency and behavioral development. *American Journal of Clinical Nutrition* 50(supplement):565–705, 1989.

Stoltzfus, R. Rethinking anaemia surveillance. *Lancet* 349:1764–1766, 1997.

Zhu, Yi and J. D. Haas. Iron depletion without anemia and physical performance in young women. *American Journal of Clinical Nutrition* 66(2):334–341, 1997.

FAT

American Cancer Society. Cancer Facts and Figures—1997. *www.cancer.org/statistics/*.

American Heart Association. Dietary guidelines for healthy American adults: a statement for health professionals from the nutrition committee. *Circulation* 94: 1795–1800, 1996.

Blundell, J. E. et al. Fat as a risk factor for overconsumption: satiation, satiety, and patterns of eating. *Journal of the American Dietetic Association* 97(7 suppl): s63–s69,1997.

Cotton, J. R. et al. Replacement of dietary fat with sucrose polyester: effects on energy intake and appetite control in nonobese males. *American Journal of Clinical Nutrition* 63(6):891–896, 1996.

Gatenby, Susan J. et al. Extended use of foods modified in fat and sugar content: nutritional implications in a free-living female population. *American Journal of Clinical Nutrition* 1867–1873, 1997.

Holt S. H. et al. A satiety index of common foods. *European Journal of Clinical Nutrition* Sep; 49(9):675–690, 1995.

Hu, F. B. et al. Dietary fat intake and the risk of coronary heart disease in women. *New England Journal of Medicine* 337(21):1491–1499, 1997.

Ip, C. and K. Carroll, eds. Individual fatty acids and cancer. *American Journal of Clinical Nutrition* 66(6 supplement):1505s–1581s, 1997.

Knopp, R. H. et al. Long-term cholesterol-lowering effects of 4 fat-restricted diets in hypercholesterolemic and combined hyperlidemic men—the dietary alternative study. *Journal of the American Medical Association* (18):1509–1515, 1997.

Kris-Etherton, P. M. ed. Individual fatty acids and cardiovascular disease. *American Journal of Clinical Nutrition* 65(5 Supplement):1577s–1699s, 1997.

Kris-Etherton, P. M. ed. Trans fatty acids and coronary heart disease risk-report of the expert panel on trans fatty acids and coronary heart diseases. *American Journal of Clinical Nutrition* 62(3 supplement):655s–708s, 1995.

Rivlin, R. S. Fats and oil in consumption in health and disease. *American Journal of Clinical Nutrition* 66(4 supplement):959s–1060s, 1997.

Siguel, E. N. and R. H. Lerman. Role of essential fatty acids: dangers in the U.S. Department of Agriculture's dietary recommendations ("pyramid") and in low-fat diets. *American Journal of Clinical Nutrition* (60):973–974, 1994.

Williams, C. L. and G. M. Williams. Reducing dietary fat: putting theory into practice. *Journal of the American Dietetic Association* 97(7 supplement):s5–s96, 1997.